This book contains a treasure trove of creative ideas and suggestions based on Joan's extensive experience and knowledge of working firstly as a social worker for many years and then as a dramatherapist and play therapist, supporting adoptive, foster and kinship parents, and placing creative play, drama and storytelling at the centre of her work with children

Clive Holmwood, Associate Professor &
Dramatherapist, University of Derby

i

Therapeutic Stories for Foster, Adoptive and Kinship Families

This accessible resource contains therapeutic stories and guidance for adults who are supporting young people aged 10–14 in foster, adoptive or kinship families. With a solution-focused approach, the stories are designed to address a range of social and emotional problems, covering topics such as bullying, eating disorders, trauma, parents' health, homophobia and racism.

Each story is accompanied by relevant context and theory, discussion points and creative activities that will stimulate the young person's problem-solving skills and imagination, empowering them to explore solutions to situations in their own lives.

Key features include:

- 35 therapeutic stories created to help young people make sense of their experiences, illustrating empathetic responses and solutions to social and emotional difficulties.

- Discussion points and related activities based on the author's extensive practical experience and knowledge.

- Practice guidelines and case studies to illustrate how the story-making approach can be used by therapists, adoptive parents, social workers and teachers.

- Photocopiable and downloadable resources.

This book will enable foster, adoptive and kinship parents, social workers, therapists, teachers and other professionals to support the young people with whom they are working to resolve their dilemmas and enhance their self-esteem.

Joan E. Moore is an author, dramatherapist, play therapist and adoption support provider with foster, adoptive and kinship families. She works mainly in the family home, applying her "Theatre of Attachment" model of life-history therapy. Joan has written several books and articles and has completed a doctoral study at Leeds Beckett University, which focused on using story and drama to support these placements and is described in *Narrative and Dramatic Approaches to Children's*

Life Story with Foster, Adoptive and Kinship Families, published by Routledge. She supervises creative arts therapists and delivers training. Having a background in social work with children and families and Youth Justice, Joan has undertaken Expert Witness Assessments of siblings, children's care needs, parents, and assessments of prospective adoptive parents and foster and kinship carers.

Therapeutic Stories for Foster, Adoptive and Kinship Families

Addressing the Domino Effect of Issues Facing 10–14-Year-Olds

Joan E. Moore

Illustrated by Fran Taylor

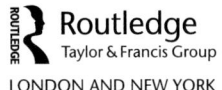

Routledge
Taylor & Francis Group

LONDON AND NEW YORK

First published 2021
by Routledge
2 Park Square, Milton Park, Abingdon, Oxon OX14 4RN

and by Routledge
52 Vanderbilt Avenue, New York, NY 10017

Routledge is an imprint of the Taylor & Francis Group, an informa business

British Library Cataloguing-in-Publication Data
A catalogue record for this book is available from the British Library

Library of Congress Cataloging-in-Publication Data
Names: Moore, Joan (Dramatherapist) author.
Title: Therapeutic stories for foster, adoptive and kinship families: addressing the domino effect of issues facing 10–14-year-olds / Joan Moore.
Description: Milton Park, Abingdon, Oxon; New York, NY: Routledge, 2021.|
Includes bibliographical references and index.
Identifiers: LCCN 2020031759 (print) | LCCN 2020031760 (ebook) |
ISBN 9780367524388 (hardback) | ISBN 9780367524371 (paperback) |
ISBN 9781003057963 (ebook)
Subjects: LCSH: Narrative therapy. |
Children with social disabilities – Counselling of.
Classification: LCC RJ505.S75 M66 2021 (print) |
LCC RJ505.S75 (ebook) | DDC 616.89/165–dc23
LC record available at https://lccn.loc.gov/2020031759
LC ebook record available at https://lccn.loc.gov/2020031760

ISBN: 978-0-367-52438-8 (hbk)
ISBN: 978-0-367-52437-1 (pbk)
ISBN: 978-1-003-05796-3 (ebk)

Typeset in Din Pro
by Newgen Publishing UK

Visit the companion website: www.routledge.com/cw/speechmark

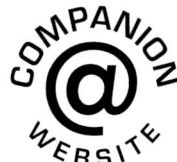

Contents

Foreword

It gives me great pleasure to write this Foreword for Joan's new book, which is a rare gift. It is rare because Joan Moore has become accomplished at bridging the gap between two worlds, the world of good theoretical reasoning with that of good practice. This book contains a treasure trove of creative ideas and suggestions based on Joan's extensive experience and knowledge of working firstly as a social worker for many years and then as a dramatherapist and play therapist, supporting adoptive, foster and kinship parents, and placing creative play, drama and storytelling at the centre of her work with children. Her previous book (Moore, 2020) describes well her "storying spiral" approach to using theatre as an attachment-based model. It is well theorised, and presents sound practical advice, as does this current book.

What Joan has done even more in this current book is to imbed theory with even greater practice, using the convention of storytelling. Ma Domino is caring and nurturing. In her domino world she takes in a range of children and young people from a range of backgrounds. Ma Domino is the kind, wise, caring, nurturing adult we would all like to be looked after by. However she is human too and admits when she doesn't always get things right. This really helps the children and young people in each story eventually to connect with her words of wisdom despite their diverse ethnic backgrounds, and family and social experiences. Ma Domino is fair, honest and non-judgemental. She sees past the children's sometimes troubling behaviours and she values the young people as they really are. It is this authenticity in Ma Domino that allows the young people to connect with her. This is what we would expect of any good enough, kinship, foster, or adoptive parent.

So who is this book for? I would argue that first and foremost this book is for foster, adoptive and kinship parents. Having worked in this sector for many years I have noticed that we are constantly extolling the importance of therapeutic parenting, without always explaining what we mean by this and more importantly supporting foster and adoptive parents to work in this way. This often leaves these vital carers with a lack of confidence in their own innate skills and abilities. Joan's earlier work (2020) reveals the importance of the therapist working with the foster and adoptive carers. This book emphasises the vital importance of this role in supporting the young people, whom ironically the carers know best, better than any professional, as the caregivers are living with the young people in their homes 24 hours a day.

The other rather sad thing to note is that, due to the ever-increasing erosion in services over the last few years and a lack of therapy and educational professionals trained in special needs, more often than not this aspect of therapeutic parenting is falling back on fostering, kinship and adoptive carers. So often I have heard these very same carers say, "I'm not a therapist", "I don't want to do or say the wrong thing", "I am not trained", "I don't want to open a can of worms", "I don't have the skills", and "I haven't been given any training". All of this is of course sadly, often true. We should not and do not expect the caregiver to take on the role of an educator, therapist or social worker. Ironically, foster carers often complain they are described as being professionals with one breath and then not with another, depending on the context or situation, which many find frustrating and irritating.

The caregivers often ask "So what is my role then?" What we can do is support them to feel more confident about their role and how they might work in safe, distanced and discreet ways to support the emotional well-being of the young people in their care. This book does exactly that. Not every parent will feel confident or especially comfortable to use these stories in the ways it describes but at the very least this book will give them a chance to understand narrative approaches already used by many other professionals. It will introduce them to the notion of using stories as a way of distancing children from the complex difficulties many of them will have experienced. It might also be useful to discuss with a therapist or social worker, which stories might be worth working on with a young person, although the carer should ultimately decide if this is right. However the stories and the structure in this book provide solid theoretical, practical and creative ideas to use with children and young people in a safe, practical, creative and most importantly, fun way.

Secondly this book is also for a range of other professionals, teachers and teaching assistants, social workers and therapists. All of these professionals may use the ideas in this book slightly differently. For example in an educational setting teachers might find these stories useful with an individual child or as a discussion point within a health and social care context within a class. Many of the issues are relevant to so many young people today. Therapists may use the stories as an on-going part of their therapy work with a child and parent. The therapist will have the skills to potentially work at a deeper level and longer term, and may or may not connect the stories directly with the child's personal experiences – something some teachers or foster carers may find too difficult. A social worker, who is specially trained in direct work, may use the stories in relation to life-story work (as might a therapist) in helping a child to reach an improved understanding of their past experiences, but again some caregivers might be less confident of undertaking this delicate task.

Whatever your background, you will hopefully be able to use this book and the many cleverly written stories, host of discussion points and creative ideas to slowly, but surely, in a non-judgemental way, just like Ma Domino does, gain the trust and provide a listening ear to the complex dilemmas and difficulties that many children in foster, kinship or adoptive families are facing. Long may this creative, gentle, caring work continue and be led by some the most important "essential" workers in our society, including the care-giving parents, with some of the most vulnerable children and young people, who are or who have been in the care system.

Dr Clive Holmwood
Associate Professor & Dramatherapist
Department of Therapeutic Arts
University of Derby
April 2020

Reference

Moore, J. (2020) *Narrative and Dramatic Approaches to Children's Life Story with Foster, Adoptive and Kinship Families: Using the Theatre of Attachment Model.* London: Routledge

Acknowledgements

Firstly, I would like to thank the foster, adoptive and kinship parents and children, who have been the inspiration for these stories. I have taken care to protect their confidentiality and be sensitive to cultural issues. Thank you to the social workers – advocates for this intervention and so appreciative.

I am grateful to Dr Clive Holmwood for his generosity in writing the foreword to his book and his helpful advice. I am also indebted to my gifted colleague Fran Taylor, art therapist, for her wonderful illustrations, as well as to my therapy colleagues, Nicky Dyer, Penny McFarlane, Claire McKenzie, and Fiona Peacock for their positive feedback and support.

Huge thanks are also due to Clare Ashworth, Senior Editor at Speechmark, and the publishing team at Routledge for their faith in this book. Last but not least, I thank my husband, children and their partners, and my extended family and friends for their enduring love and valued encouragement.

Introduction

Why is the book needed?

This collection of stories is primarily for young people, aged 10–14, who are living in foster, adoptive and kinship families. The aim is to help them acquire the insight and self-confidence to deal with their emotional problems and access the support they need. Feelings are intrinsic to our lives as they affect our physical well-being and influence how we think, understand and relate to the world around us. Emotional, mental and physical maturity varies considerably between 10 and 14 years of age. Children's relationships with their peers and caregivers can be further complicated by social and media influences on top of the traumatic experiences of neglect and abuse that so many will have experienced. Increasingly, in the wake of rising poverty and reduced public funding, the agencies supporting children and their families are seeing an alarming rise in mental illness especially in this age group.

NHS statistics (*Independent*, 9 January 2020) report the numbers of Looked After Children, who are self-harming to be double those of children in the general population referred for this reason. The impact of social isolation prompted by the 2020 Coronavirus pandemic will have left many of these children experiencing disconnection from their friends and support systems. The high numbers of deaths prolonging the lockdown alongside financial worries affecting many families have exacerbated the children's trauma and anxieties.

Who can use this book?

While the stories and activities are mainly aimed at children and their adoptive, foster and kinship parents, they can also be used with individuals and small groups in the general population. For example, support staff in pupil referral units and children's homes might read a story as a way of talking about an issue affecting a child or small group. Trained therapists in clinical and school settings or in the family home could use the stories to explore the children's experiences at a deeper level. Many of the stories will also be useful to social workers for exploring the children's feelings in preparation for life-story work. The stories and worksheets can also be accessed from the website at: www.routledge.com/cw/speechmark in order that they can be photocopied for sharing with the child. Chapter 7 gives practice guidelines and four case studies to illustrate how therapists, adoptive parents, social workers and teachers can apply this story-making approach. Sunderland (2015) gives valuable guidance on drawing out children's feelings. While acknowledging that many adults worry about not having adequate training to address children's feelings, I strongly believe that showing sensitivity, genuine interest and giving your time can go a long way to helping children feel listened to and cared about.

The issues addressed

The stories are designed to help the children make sense of their experiences since enhancing their understanding of self and others enables them to gain more from life. Set on the imaginary "Planet Domino", named after the "domino effect" of each event having an impact on the next, the stories feature problems arising from the traumas of neglect and abuse, domestic violence, parents' substance addiction, mental ill-health, bullying, racism, disability, female genital mutilation, forced child marriage, self-harm and loss. The purpose of the creative activities is to invite the children to explore their feelings in sufficient depth that they feel heard and gain a sense of empowerment. Though many issues are not so easily "fixed" in real life, the brevity of these stories makes them easier to adapt and tailor to individual need, for example by allowing the young person to decide how a story might be continued. Care needs to be taken with children's privacy and dignity. Distressed children who feel unsupported or misunderstood have to be able to trust their care-giving parents more than anyone else. Neuroscience research finds the key to inviting positive change to lie in attuning to emotions. It is therefore very important to create opportunities to talk about feelings and enable children to express their negative ones of anger and distress, which are just as important as their positive feelings.

These stories can be used to help children make wiser decisions that protect them from entrapment. The positive solutions convey a sense of hope. Issues such as cyber-bullying, game addiction, self-harm and social isolation are affecting progressively more children, especially the most vulnerable. Fictional privacy renders it unnecessary for the adult to delve into the child's problems in the way that therapy can. The stories and activities provide a springboard to invite children to explore the social and moral issues affecting them today and find their own solutions, which may not always be those illustrated in the story.

Positive feelings of fun, laughter and excitement are enormously important because they stimulate the production of neural chemicals, which help to protect the brain from the deleterious effects of depression and anxiety.

Method

The method is built on the Storying Spiral (Moore, 2019), founded on the arousal-attachment cycle (Fahlberg, 1994, 2008). In this cycle, the child expresses a need that on being met enables him or her to be confident this will continue. The parent or practitioner working with the child selects the story they think the child will connect to. After hearing the story, the child is encouraged to engage in the accompanying creative activities. Praise and deep listening from the attentive adult will inspire the child to create their own story and to re-engage in the exercise in future opportunities. This cycle repeats, gradually moving into a spiral as the children find their own solutions and come to need less support. Provision of creative materials invites the child to use the materials as they wish – to play and/or develop stories in their own way.

The adult's task is to reflect on the action and feelings they perceive to be arising in the child's play: "This one is hiding – is she scared? Does she need help?" Adopting the enthusiastic manner of a sports commentator, you might say, "Wow, how exciting! This guy is so brave!" Conveying a warm, enthusiastic manner will help children to feel appreciated. The discussion points, followed by reflections, provide a guide for the safe exploration of feelings via keeping mainly to the story's content, as detailed in Chapter 7. It might take more than one session to explore a topic since the activities can arouse strong feelings. Typing and illustrating emerging stories makes them more accessible to reread. It also reinforces the children's learning and enhances their self-esteem.

Safe practice

The issues raised in the stories are important to discuss. Even so, the highly sensitive content makes it important to ensure privacy for the child. The adult is therefore guided to talk about the characters in the stories rather than to directly question individuals, who may not feel safe to disclose their feelings in that moment. Children, who have been bullied, need to know there is someone they can safely confide in. However, allegations of abuse must be acted on in accordance with safeguarding policy. Collaboration with involved adults is important, to ensure support and avoid risk of confusion or conflict.

Although there is huge variation in maturity between the ages of 10 and 14, many of the issues addressed in this book are affecting children at a younger age. In any case, children are often aware of their older siblings' problems, and for their own protection, will benefit from preparation for future challenges by gaining an improved understanding of these issues and ways to stay safe.

How the book is laid out

Themes inevitably, overlap, but are grouped under the chapter headings of:

(1) Family tensions (2) Trauma abuse and neglect (3) The legacy of mental illness, (4) Social, emotional and mental health needs, (5) Difference and isolation, and (6) Social media pressures. Each chapter features topics related to its title and contains a summary of the issues and ideas on how to support the children. Following each of the stories are suggested creative activities and a set of discussion points to invite exploration of feelings. Further reflections are provided to help the adult to respond to children's questions and explore their arising feelings.

Stories – a tool for problem solving

Stories provide a wonderful escape from the grim realities of life. When carefully chosen, they bring joy, satisfaction and knowledge, all of which enhance a sense of well-being. Since time immemorial, stories and their symbols have been enhancing our spirituality and imagination (Warner, 2014). Indeed Harari (2014) extols that historically, stories are the means by which communities have built on shared beliefs – we humans have survived via cooperation and persuasion and organised ourselves by devising scripts and hierarchies, which are the product of human imagination.

Drawing from the emergence of language and culture, Boyd (2018) cites extensive evidence of the crucial role that stories have played in evolution. Stories enable humans to imagine the future and prepare for it by re-evaluating experience from new perspectives. Boyd points out that as a story reveals what is affecting the central character's attempts to achieve a difficult goal, we want to know what happens next and how the characters in the story change as a result.

Story plots

Stories of heroes' survival of adversity often have special appeal to emotionally burdened children. Booker (2004) identified seven basic story plots, which follow a pattern whereby the main character moves from a state of dependency towards independence. Fictional heroes such as Odysseus exemplify the individual's need for a 'secure base' (Bowlby, 1989) to return to, before they feel ready to explore the world. For characters in *The Wonderful Wizard of Oz* and *Peter Pan*, transportation to another world parallels the experience for children removed from their families of origin to foster care and adoption. The heroes often make mistakes but through sheer endurance they achieve their goal, thereby giving hope to the anxious young reader. In the story of *Hansel and Gretel*, the witch is projected as an insensitive, sometimes, terrorising force. Her lack of understanding is symbolic of human imperfection. Despite this, the young heroes manage to outwit her. The fairy stories *Cinderella* and *Aladdin* characterise the transformation from miserable dejection to desired fulfilment.

It is the magnifying of emotion in the fictional context that enables a better understanding of reality. A benefit of dramatising these tales is the taking on of fictional roles as this enables children to adapt to new ways of thinking and new perspectives. The process helps them to communicate their thoughts more effectively and enjoy the positive consequences. It is a specific form of healing theatre that Jennings (2012) views as a "rite of passage" through emotional distress to facilitate the journey from unwell-being to well-being.

Creating stories

Children are often reluctant to talk directly about their problems. As stories such as "Dukha's secret" in Chapter 5 illustrate, the fictional context makes it easier for a young person to admit to the need to share worries or put wrongs right. This is because the act of creating a story enhances the connections between the "emotional" right and the "rational" left hemispheres of the brain via the emerging metaphors. Metaphors such as "swimming against the tide" and "being crushed underfoot" serve as a bridge, connecting feelings and experience. In this process, children make links between cause and effect as they rationalise the past and discover new possibilities for the future.

Coholic (2010) found the process of creating narratives led children aged 8 to 13 years to explore their spirituality and imagination. In this process they find meaning to actions in what might otherwise seem a meaningless universe. The distancing effect of projective work with story, dolls, puppets and images is particularly helpful to working with powerful emotions (Moore et al., 2017).

Creating narratives is the foundation of my work, helping children of all ages to make sense of disruption in their lives (Moore, 2012; 2014; 2020). Stories of heroes undergoing adversity invite the children to identify with the character's feelings of

5

rejection, loss and betrayal, yet as it is "just" a story, children are free to accept, refute or ignore its connection to their own experience.

Accessing the senses

The sensory mediums of art, drama, poetry and music are among the many different ways in which emotional problems can be worked through. Neuroscience increasingly demonstrates the importance of play for enhancing human development (Panksepp, 2015). Beckoff explains that creative play "provides important nourishment for brain growth; it actually helps to rewire the brain, increasing connections between neurons in the cerebral cortex" (2007, 100). The process of experimenting with natural materials often brings unconscious feelings to conscious awareness. As children see their creations turn into another form that has different properties – such as clay that starts wet then dries – subconsciously they learn that the possibilities of change also apply to them. In engaging the senses, creative activities allow feelings to be processed at a deeper level than is possible from just talking about them.

Enabling new insights

During late childhood as theory of mind develops (Kokkinos et al., 2015) young people learn subtler ways of extending and linking events. Sutton-Smith (1981) noticed that pre-adolescents' stories became more active, resourceful and resolute with well-formed episodes and continuity. By this age, children are incorporating their aims, intentions, feelings and beliefs, at first implicitly, then explicitly into their own stories and their responses to questions about the stories they've read. Imagination transports us to other spheres of existence and allows us to explore not just what is known to be true but what *might* be true or *could* have occurred. In fictional contexts, magic is a device for contriving desired outcomes until the child is ready to conceive of realistic ways forward. Boyd (2009) remarks that stories facilitate our understanding of social situations in real life by improving our capacity to interpret events and "to shift mentally to new characters, times, and perspectives" (p. 193).

Family relationships

Chapter 1 focuses on the plight of children in foster, kinship and adoptive families, who have lost the stories that ensure a sense of identity gained from knowing who they are and where they came from. The legacy of neglect and trauma poses huge challenges to relationships. Raby and Dozier (2019) note that while adoption has enabled the most traumatised children to make remarkable recovery, adverse care has long-lasting repercussions on their attachment relationships and on their adoptive parents' attachment representations. Too often when trust has been betrayed, the children will continue to struggle to trust in any future caregivers. Patterns of insecure and disorganised attachment prompting avoidance, ambivalence or a combination of both, can disrupt these parents' best efforts to care for their children. Although traumatic neglect and abuse severely compromise the child's ability to form a secure attachment, the story "Darma's despair" illustrates how repair can be achieved. Debate continues as to the relevant influence of genes and environment on survival of adverse beginnings. The stories in this chapter reflect on the impact of disrupted care, pressures of sibling rivalries, conflict and divided loyalties, and conclude with one on social isolation to illustrate the impact of lockdown and ways to mitigate its deleterious effects.

Brain development

Chapter 2 focuses on the child's experience of trauma, neglect and abuse. The stories address topics of neglect, verbal and sexual abuse, memory problems, foetal alcohol effect, school phobia and hiding. To make sense of the ways in which abuse and trauma alongside today's social and media influences affect this age group, let us consider how the pre-teen brain develops. It used to be assumed that the brain was fully-grown by adolescence. Now we know that in late childhood the volume of "grey matter" peaks and decreases at the start of puberty. At this stage the volume of white matter increases, enhancing speed and decision-making into adulthood. Waters et al. (2019) describe early adolescence as a pivotal period of development in which parents play a key role in their child's mental health. Throughout adolescence, huge changes take place in a child's physical appearance and identity, as well as their social life and relationships.

Curiously 10-year-olds are often found to have greater capacity for empathy than 13-year-olds. One explanation for this phenomenon is that the brain parts responsible for expressing emotions and seeking reward mature earlier than those, which oversee careful decision-making and impulse control. While this is likely to be at least partly true, some challenge the claims that unique changes occur in the brain during adolescence and maintain that often the young person's environment has far greater influence on how they get on through the teenage years. Of course at this stage there is a lot to learn and the sheer bombardment of new stimuli takes time to assimilate. But when 12- and 13-year-olds argue compulsively, appear volatile, clumsy or to be taking too many unsafe risks, this is at least partially attributable to external factors such as family disharmony, exam stress and media pressures.

Decision-making

Early in adolescence, young people do not have the maturity or independence to be able to weigh up multiple and conflicting information, a task made even more difficult when their development has been delayed by abuse or neglect.

At the front part of the upper cortex (also referred to as the "executive" brain) the pre-frontal cortex (or forebrain) is responsible for the planning and insight required to formulate strategies, inhibit impulses and guide decision-making and is reorganising at around 11–14 years. At this age, brain scans reveal the young person to be susceptible to acute self-consciousness when they anticipate others are judging them (Blakemore, 2018). Indeed Frydenburgh (2008) found young people of this age to be more anxious than older teenagers about making decisions and less likely to seek the support they need. The pre-teens fretted about the wider effect of their decisions and not just important ones; they experienced stress in making even everyday decisions about what to wear, which TV programme to watch and how to repair a friendship.

Risk-taking

The route to independence inevitably involves taking risks. After all, young people need to learn to make their own decisions. In adolescence, risk-taking peaks as friends (and the need to impress them) become more important than at any other stage in life. Risk-taking and sensation seeking can be especially fraught for children and their foster, adoptive or kinship parents. Usually when faced with scenes of deliberate actions and their consequences, feelings are brought to awareness and rationalised by the upper brain. But the brains of traumatised young people rely far longer on the amygdala – the part that galvanises "fight-flight-freeze" reactions to threat. Risk-taking activates dopamine, the neurotransmitter responsible for generating feelings of thrill and assisting emotional regulation. However too much dopamine desensitises the brain and leaves the child such as "Dotty" – Story 8 – craving to repeat the thrill. It means that at the age of 10–14, these young people are even more reliant on safe boundaries and emotional support from parents and teachers.

Flexibility

Lehrer describes the human brain as more flexible than rational – "like a computer operating system with design flaws and software bugs that was rushed to market" (Lehrer, 2009, 24). Yet the delay in forebrain completion heightens flexibility, which arguably, makes young people's brains powerful precisely because as "work in progress" they are so receptive to experience. Frydenburgh (2008) examined gender differences between 11–14-year-olds and found the teaching of problem-solving methods effective for reducing self-blame in both genders. Certainly in my experience, if we want children to talk about the issues affecting them, rather than focus on a child's specific problem, children will engage more readily in discussion on the effect of actions and consequences affecting fictional characters.

Heightened sensitivity

The stage of preparing for independence often brings associated angst. The stories in this book illustrate the huge significance of peer influences on pre-teen children, who, due to past rejection, tend to self-blame and be especially sensitive to disapproval. Anticipating further rejection, many are all too ready to believe criticism and depend heavily on their friends' approval. They rely on adults to model how to cope maturely with disappointments. Losses of attachment relationships disrupt memory systems, which usually allow us to take the routines and habits of life for granted. Ordinarily, the brain makes connections between the senses that alert us (so for example, if we hear our phone ring we instinctively look for it) but distressing loss interferes in this process. The story of "Dilly" in Chapter 2 demonstrates how it can leave the child confused. Neglect early in life means that difficulties in recognising social signals such as nods and hints, implicit knowledge that most of us take for granted impedes the child's skill in communication. Indeed Mehrabium (2017) estimates non-verbal aspects of communication to be as high as 80%.

Chapter 3 on the legacy of mental illness illustrates the predicaments of children and young people exposed to domestic violence, living with mentally ill parents, suffering post-traumatic stress, low self-esteem and showing self-harming behaviour such as eating disorder. Without appropriate support, the strain of these predicaments can easily overwhelm these young people.

Illustrating the plight of an asylum-seeking young person suffering post-traumatic stress disorder (PTSD), the story "Dixie's devastation" explains that in some cultures it would be regarded as disrespectful for her to look adults in the eye (Caw and Sebba, 2014). In other cultures in which eye contact conveys respect, the avoidance of eye contact can lead to misunderstandings. Adoptive, foster and kinship parents can enable their children to recognise the subtle variations in expressions of emotion by encouraging more face-to-face interaction with their friends.

Recognition of emotions in others is an important part of emotion processing. Hunnikin et al. (2019) found children at risk of involvement in criminal activities to be significantly impaired in recognising emotions in faces, especially fear and sadness. According to De Heering et al. (2012) children's recognition of facial expression improves between 6 and 12 years and is more enhanced after age 12, particularly for upright faces. Eye contact may be used to elicit cooperation or be a means of exercising social control by expressing intimacy or threat. This helps to explain why young people in foster, kinship and adoptive families can find eye contact with adults so tricky.

Changing social trends

In contemporary times, fewer children are playing outdoors in the fresh air. Nairn (2011), on finding less than 33% of (all) children engaging in the adventurous play enjoyed by 70% in the previous generation saw a correlating rise in mental illness and bullying. An inadvertent risk in restricting pre-teens from unsupervised outdoor play may be greater exposure to other risks such as involvement with chat rooms, porn and online gaming, risks they are not equipped or ready to deal with, as illustrated in Chapter 6.

Chapter 4, concerned with social, emotional and mental health needs, reflects on the plight of young people for whom selective mutism, autism, dyspraxia, attention deficit hyperactivity disorder (ADHD), dyslexia and living with an alcoholic parent has left them vulnerable to bullying, exclusion and addiction.

These problems frequently coincide with others such as PTSD and mean that under stress the child's amygdala is activated to remind them they are in danger. The child, who has moved many times expects rejection and may act to "get in first" and act in a rejecting way to protect themselves from anticipated disappointment, unable to believe that they might actually be wanted. A story that illustrates the predicament of the children with alcoholic parents is "Dusty's distress", a story to convey that affected children can be helped to feel better supported and prepared.

Difference and isolation

Chapter 5 begins with reflection on the anxiety-inducing effects of the intimidation aroused in instances of racism, homophobia and sexism. It illustrates the importance of giving voice to the victims and goes on to illustrate the safeguarding concerns of female genital mutilation (FGM) and forced child marriage, described in the last two stories. The Knowledge Hub provides access to guidance, research and practice of FGM. On finding that 170,000 girls under 15 had undergone this procedure, Bindel (2014) explains the need for cultural sensitivity in the use of language for trying to encourage more enlightened attitudes. The term "female genital cutting" is more neutral and less politicised but the DfE report (2017) adopts the term FGM to acknowledge the severity of harm it causes, as illustrated in "Dukha's secret". The report's authors find FGM to frequently co-present with forced child marriage, which is widely considered to be child abuse, although not in traditional cultures in which parental rights justify it (Kopelman, 2016). In the exploitation of girls being threatened, deceived, coerced into compliance and treated as property, there is an overlap with slavery (Vidal, 2016), as described in "Drina and Dilip's drama".

The impact of social media

Chapter 6 focuses on social media pressures given that there has never been a more pressing need for vulnerable children to receive help to make sense of the situations in which they find themselves. Social media is permeating every aspect of our daily lives and is changing patterns of interaction with family and friends. The Internet and social media platforms provide new ways of learning as well as enhanced connectivity. Since the start of enforced lockdown, it has been proving especially useful. Even so we cannot afford to ignore the risks and detrimental effects that social media can have on the most vulnerable children in foster, kinship and adoptive families.

Children and young people now have the agency to create a level of privacy and self-development that is out of sight and reach of their parents, caregivers and other adults such as teachers, who are responsible for their safety. The ease with which a child can set up profiles on sites such as Instagram and Snapchat means they gate-keep and restrict access to their information. It also makes it easier for them to threaten and cause distress to anyone they choose to target as illustrated in the story, "Decision for Dana", Chapter 6.

Ehmke (2019) alerts us to the child's compulsion to focus on a small screen to keep up with gossip and avoid being left out. Children and adolescents often fear falling out with their friends if they are not quick enough in responding to them (Sen, 2015). This trend has reduced their opportunity to practise social signals and interpret others' feelings. Children's brains depend on face-to-face interactions to learn how to communicate effectively and social isolation is not helping. A concern is that the more children give in to technology – texts, updates and games – the less connected and extensive their neural circuits will be for focusing on tasks and sustaining attention. The story "Dariel's obsession" in Chapter 6 describes a young person's fixation with online gaming and illustrates how he is encouraged to take up new interests.

Earlier maturation and the lessening of taboo about sex gives young people more power than ever to make their own decisions but leaves girls vulnerable to being persuaded to have sex before they are physically and emotionally ready. Sen (2015) quotes from young people's accounts indicating that sexual objectivity of girls and young women works alongside long-standing social constructions of sexual activity as a highly positive sign of status for boys and a highly negative one for girls. Sales (2016) finds girls being lured to upload compromising photos that get shared indiscriminately with devastating consequences.

This emphasises the need for filtering software to reduce harm from likely risk to reputation, sexual predators, cyber-bullying and to screen time and online gaming. The stories in this chapter promote ways of engaging the young people in activities that will help to keep them safer. Still Simpson (2016) warns that a danger of scrutinising children's certain behaviours is that the adults can easily misinterpret the child's online conversation due to their lack of awareness of the context. It is incredibly important for care-giving parents, teachers and social workers to talk with young people about the risks they may be taking and to familiarise themselves with how the social media platforms work and how the risks may effectively be mitigated. Chapter 7 provides guidance and case studies to enable adults in this important task.

Assessment

It is important to take account of past impact on the child's current, (possibly trauma-induced) reactions and to note:

- What may be triggering worrying incidents.
- The quality of the child's relationships.
- The child's language skill and understanding of what you say to them.
- The child's stage (not just age) of emotional and cognitive development.
- How the child copes with praise e.g. dismisses or views with suspicion.
- The cultural expectations of the child and their foster/adoptive/kinship family, which may differ from each other.

Next, let me introduce the cast of people on Planet Domino.

Planet Domino

Planet Domino could be thought of as a fictional planet in outer space, which took the overspill when Earth became too densely populated. Or it might be the name of a housing estate anywhere. Domino people vary in appearance: They can be rounded or straight, black or white, plain or colourfully adorned. The first arrivals to Planet Domino had already experienced the disastrous consequences of social unrest. Having witnessed the "domino effect" of each event on the next, they named their community "Planet Domino" and built houses rather like the "boxes" in which domino pieces are packaged. The Dominos worked together to build a community, which continues to expand.

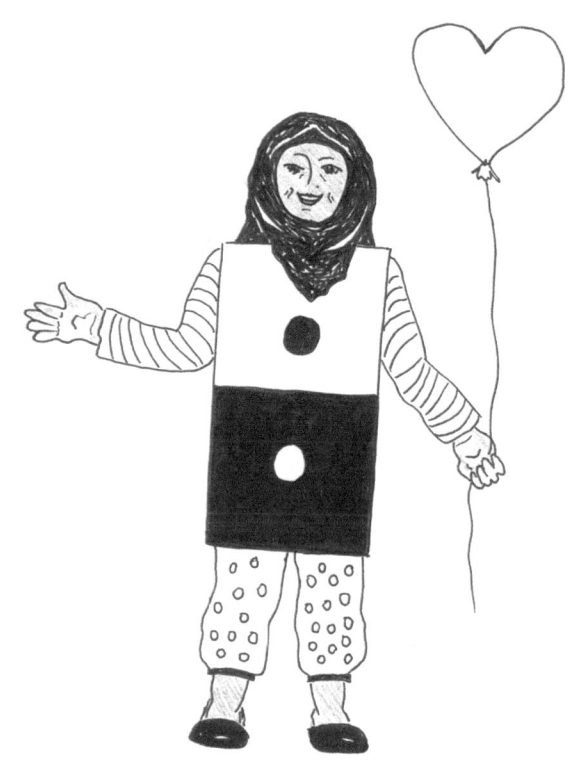

On this planet is a household headed by Ma Domino, whose partner died some years ago, leaving her with no money. She decided to open her home to vulnerable young people in need of shelter and care. In the stories to follow, her adoptive and foster children aged between 10 and 14 all need her help.

As occurs universally, the young domino characters in these stories have encountered parental' depression, illness, addiction and disability. Social and media influences bring further pressures, and for those subjected to ignorant attitudes and bullying, an additional sense of social isolation and inadequacy. An experienced mother figure, Ma Domino dispenses wisdom as she patiently uses every tool at her disposal to help the young dominoes in her care to discover their strengths and gain the confidence to resolve matters for themselves, and feel supported to achieve their ambitions.

1 Family tensions

New family relationships

Family relationships are the way we first learn about reciprocity and cooperation – they are the "glue" that secures our sense of belonging. It is the quality of these relationships, which determines children's mental health and happiness. When attachment has been disrupted, children can lose trust in adults' ability to keep them safe and cared for.

In their family of origin, children will have used survival strategies to get their needs met. These strategies often perpetuate in the new family and may be experienced by foster, kinship and adoptive parents as overly coercive or rejecting and therein discouraging of their efforts. The children's continued use of the strategies is instinctive. The reason for this is that their neural alarm system has become accustomed to surviving abuse and neglect, which their brains expect to continue. It is why the most traumatised children and young people need professional help to process their earlier experience and reconstruct their behaviour as that of heroic survival.

Children, who have not received the quality of attention they needed from (birth) parents, frequently have fraught relationships with their siblings, each competing to undermine the other's needs in order to get their own met. It can leave the new parents exhausted as they try to accommodate the needs of all their children. Indeed Selwyn (2019) found that siblings placed together were statistically more likely to disrupt than sequential placements. Only 18 out of the 83 families in her study described normal sibling relationships.

On reaching adolescence young people begin to seek greater independence. At this stage the complexity around contact with birth families and access to social media may further compromise their safety. The child's first loyalty is so often to the parents they were born to. The child may assume it is impossible to love both sets of parents without showing disloyalty to one or the other. Kim and Tucker (2019) remark that complex dynamics are inherent in navigating these often, ambiguous relationships – not least concerns about safety. In the processes involved in contact with birth family, foster and adoptive families, Fuentes et al. (2018) find key problems are lack of preparation and support.

A recent issue affecting adopted and fostered young people reaching the stage of seeking greater independence, is the lockdown restrictions imposed to stop the spread of the Coronavirus. For many, fears about their own and their caregivers' health and well-being as well as being isolated from their friends and school have only added to their anxiety.

The stories in this chapter illustrate the complex feelings of children caught up in family disruption, including conflict with their care-giving parents, sibling rivalry and co-dependence, problematic contact with their birth family and surviving enforced social isolation. These stories illustrate ways to help children to process their experience and find new ways forward.

Family disruption

In the UK, nearly 50% of families break up and reconstituted families have become commonplace. While many single families and stepfamilies are successful, the course of renegotiating relationships can cause the children to experience anger, resentment and anxiety. The stories in this chapter address anxieties arising from conflict, divided loyalties, sibling rivalry and lockdown in adoptive and foster families consequent to the children's experience of neglect and disruption in their previous families, including foster placements.

In Story 1, Dora is tired of the bickering between members of her family. On moving to Ma Domino's, she is helped to think of ways to share resources that will alleviate the pressure and enable her to reconcile to her new situation.

How to use this story

- Read the story and use the discussion points to explore the children's perceptions of parents and children's own responsibilities.

- Discuss positive ways to address Dora's anxieties.

- Encourage practice at dealing maturely with conflict.

- Prepare children to act responsibly when adults are not around.

- Through the creative activities, invite the children to explore the pros and cons of possible resolutions to conflicts and how to negotiate them.

- Help anxious children find activities and outlets that will give them social support and respite from their worries.

Story 1: Dora's dilemma

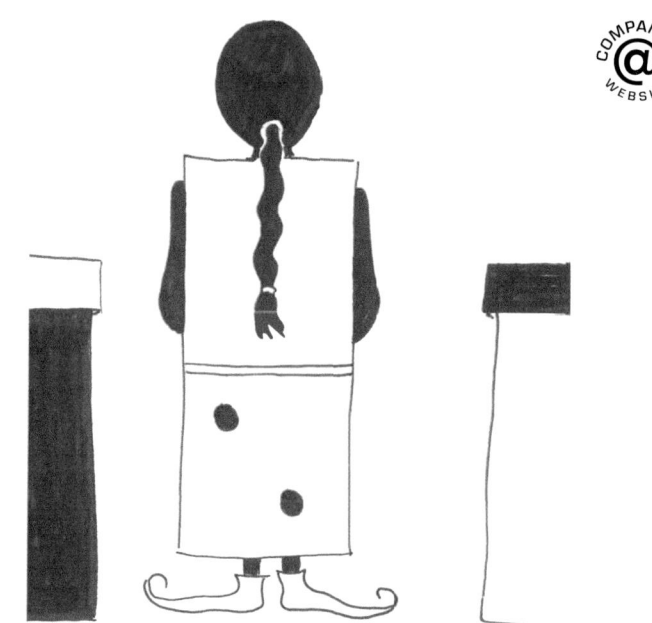

Dora's family had split up and her parents were living with their new partners. Dora, aged 12, and her 10-year-old brother stayed at their Dad's and the youngest two stayed at Mum's. Both their stepparents had children living with them. They all bickered as they resented getting less attention from their parents, who seemed to mainly shout at them. For Dora, sharing her life between the two families meant being carted from one place to another and frequently losing her stuff along the way. Living part of the week in each household had got horribly confusing. Dora had to keep trying to remember which day of the week it was and where she was supposed to be. It felt like she didn't have a proper home any more. Her stepparents no longer seemed to like Dora or her brothers and sister. Dad started drinking and Dora's brother told his teacher about it. Dora was furious with him when the social workers took them to Ma Domino's place.

Luckily Ma Domino seemed to understand how difficult things were for Dora, who said, "It's like being in two half finished jigsaws with pieces missing or not matching!" Nodding sympathetically Ma said, "That reminds me!" She went to the cupboard to fetch boxes of jigsaws she'd collected with the aim of distracting her charges away from their small screens. Ma Domino explained, "These puzzles are all mixed up – will you help me sort them out?" As they made up the jigsaws, Ma Domino encouraged Dora to figure out good things about having a brother and sister and stepsiblings. Dora found it helped to have a grownup listen carefully and show genuine interest in her. It got her thinking about the things they missed. She worked out that some of the skates in Dad's garage could be swapped for footballs at Mum's. As she got used to living at Ma Domino's, Dora grew fonder of her brothers, sister and stepsisters, whom she saw at school. When they had a problem, they came to her to talk it over and together they'd find a solution.

Activities

- Make a jigsaw by drawing and painting a family scene on to card. (Or find a clip art scene, print it and glue it onto card.) Turn the card over and draw jigsaw shapes on the reverse side and cut out these shapes.

- In pairs, think about ways to take turns, share spaces and equipment.

- Discuss sharing systems that work and what happens when they don't.

- Make a list of games and activities for families to enjoy.

Materials

Stiff card, paper, crayons, pens, scissors, craft knives.

Discussion

- What bothers Dora most about her life? Whom could she talk to?

- In new families it can be difficult to share the space, time and attention. What is it like to share a bedroom with a sibling you've only recently met? How can foster and adoptive parents make it easier?

- Is coping with moving, especially into foster care stressful, and as Dora found, does it mean you have even more rules to learn and remember?

- Think of the different sensory experiences. Have you noticed different smells in each house you've lived in? Is one house tidier? How do the differences in each place you've lived in affect you?

- What do you think the next chapter of the story might be? Will Dora stay with Ma Domino or move home? What might be the outcome?

Reflections

- Going between two households meant that Dora missed the stability of living in one place. She hated losing things and forgetting which house she'd left them in. Dora was also tired of the squabbling going on between her siblings, parents and their partners. Perhaps what Dora most missed was being settled and having fewer worries.

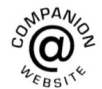

- To support children in this situation, parents could arrange a time to give each child individual attention to show them their feelings matter. Sharing a bedroom, especially with a new sibling, is rarely easy. It takes lots of negotiation to agree what can be shared without ill feeling.

- Each house tends to have its own smell. Cooking smells reflect culture and tradition. Everyone has their own ideas on tidiness and hygiene and everyone thinks they've got it right. For children, moving to a new family inevitably presents challenges. Having to get used to all the changes is likely to cause disorientation and confusion.

- Talking over these changes and the effects they are having will help to prevent and ameliorate the build up of distress and anxiety. Some children, who arrive in care, will have been accustomed to far greater freedom than their foster and adoptive parents will feel able to allow, due to having responsibilities for keeping children safe.

- Acknowledging children's feelings and giving reassurance and clear explanations about the reason for rules, as frequently as necessary, will help children to feel accepted. They may need an identified adult at school whom they can talk to about their feelings.

Divided loyalties

In recent years, unemployment and low pay have been affecting the lifestyle of increasingly more families, reducing income for basic clothes, outings and treats, which they might once have taken for granted. In 2019, the End Child Poverty Coalition[BIB-025] reported that over 54% of children in the UK were living in poverty, a rise testified by the huge spread of food banks and is even more exacerbated by the impact of lockdown and job losses. The stress this causes often leads to depression, and sometimes further disruption and greater financial hardship. For a proportion of families, conflicts lead to the children being taken into care. For young people aged 10–14 it can feel very important to keep up with their friends' expectations, yet many repress their own needs in order to prioritise their parents' emotional well-being.

Story 2 "Dylan's dread" focuses on the anxieties affecting a young person taking on heavy responsibilities for his struggling family.

How to use this story

- Read the story and discuss how families are being affected by poverty and unemployment. The aim is to help affected children to feel better supported and less emotionally isolated or stigmatised.

- Use the creative activity to explore what responsibilities (if any) that young people should take on when their parents are not coping well.

- Discuss ways in which young people may earn money legitimately.

Story 2: Dylan's dread

Dylan Domino, aged 13, was feeling anxious and miserable having recently moved to Ma Dominos. After his Dad lost his job, everything had started going wrong. Mum walked out as Dad got depressed and stayed in bed all day. Before long there was hardly anything to eat. If the meter ran out they went to bed early to keep warm. Dylan had holes in his shoes but he daren't ask for new ones. He took his little sisters to school then went home to wash the dishes and sort the laundry. This made him late for school. Teachers noticed his marks dipping. Dylan avoided his best mate. He just wasn't in the mood to laugh or chat about ordinary stuff. In any case it all felt too awkward to invite someone home the way things

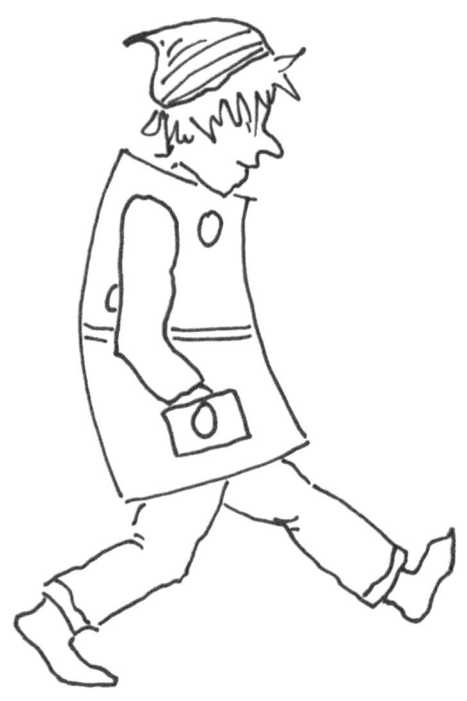

were. Then Dad met Doris. She moved in with her children, making it overcrowded. Doris said there were too many mouths to feed on her part-time wages. The row went on all night long! It ended with Doris being carted off to hospital. The next day the police took Dylan to Ma Domino's. His sisters went to a different home and he really missed them.

Dylan worried about how his Dad was coping on his own. He often popped in to check on him on the way back from school. One day as he passed a café Dylan saw his Dad inside, smiling across the table at a young woman. Dylan was shocked that Dad appeared to be spending money they didn't have. Not only that, he was chatting someone up! Dylan wondered what to do – confront Dad or pretend he hadn't noticed. It was ages since he'd seen his Dad look so happy, so he kind of dreaded spoiling it. The next day Dylan mentioned seeing him in the café. Dad replied, "it must have been someone else. I was at home all day." Dylan knew he was lying. A few days later, Dylan saw him leave the same café, so phoned Doris, who was now out of hospital. She told him his Dad had gone to a job interview. Dylan felt sick, wondering what Dad was really up to. When he got back to Ma Domino's he asked for a private word, so Ma took him into the front room. Dylan told her how scared he was that his Dad might be meeting up with another woman. Ma Domino agreed, "That sounds very worrying!" Still she reckoned he'd been wise not to accuse his father without having any definite proof. They agreed the best plan would be for Dylan to ask Dad if he'd had any luck with finding work. Ma Domino was worried about Dylan looking so pale and unhappy. She asked him what he'd enjoyed doing before all this happened. He told her about a game he and his mate had been inventing. Impressed, she said "I can think of lots of people who'd enjoy that game". Ma rang her niece Dilys, whose job was marketing games. Dilys agreed to look at selling Dylan's game when it was ready. "That's awesome!" said Dylan, thanking her. Encouraged, he called in on Dad to find him celebrating a new job serving meals at the café. The young woman he'd seen with Dad was his new boss. The money wasn't good but Dylan was massively relieved that his Dad had work and wasn't cheating on Doris. He phoned his best mate and arranged to make plans to work on their game.

Activities

- In pairs or small groups, dramatise the scene of a situation when adults are not around and you have to decide what to do. Design a board game/on-line game featuring the scene. Where can you go for advice?

- Design a leaflet advertising a service, say car washing or baking cakes.

Materials

Pens, crayons, paper and card.

Discussion

- This story had a happy outcome. What else might happen in real life?

- Dylan's Dad got depressed. Why do you think he lied to Dylan?

- Can going into foster care be harder for young people aged 10–14, than when they are younger? In what way?

- Why was Dylan late for school? What happened as a result?

- Why did Dylan think his Dad was having an affair?

- If you were in Dylan's situation where would you go for advice?

Reflections

- The reason why Dylan's Dad lied would have been to protect his son from worrying about him. His Dad was trying to get work but didn't want to overburden Dylan with his problems.

- Dylan's Dad had been depressed and was reluctant to give Dylan even more to worry about. It is a parent's job to protect children from worries as much as possible although it is also important to have mutual trust.

- At age 10–14, children begin to rely more on their friends, and to want more independence and privacy. Moving to a foster or adoptive home can mean that they lose friendships that are very important to them.

- Dylan had been late to school in order to take his sisters to school then do housework while his Dad was still in bed, having found he couldn't rely on his Dad for this. So often, children take on too much responsibility for parents, who are depressed or ill.

- Seeing his Dad in the café in the company of a young woman Dylan hadn't seen before led Dylan to jump hastily to the wrong conclusion.

- Dylan was wise to talk to Ma Domino and take her advice rather than confront his father about his fears.

Conflict with caregivers

Environment and genes both affect children's development but for adopted and fostered children the separate influences they have on outcomes are very difficult to disentangle. Sellers et al. (2019) emphasise the importance of understanding the interplay of genes and environment in order to plan intervention effectively. What is important is that since each child and family will respond differently, a "one-size-fits-all" approach is unlikely to be helpful.

Conflict in adoptive and foster families often stems from the combined factors of these parents not having a full appreciation of their child's past (often) traumatic experience, and the child being stuck in self-blame and self-hatred. What has been demonstrated as beneficial to foster, kinship and adoptive families is helping both children and parents to reach a fuller understanding of the reasons for the child's removal to care (Moore, 2020) via an empathic contextualising, which averts blame and shame of the birth parents.

Story 3: "Darma's despair" illustrates the long-term impact of early traumatic experience of physical abuse and violence on a child's learning capacity and subsequent relationships with caregivers. Problems worsen until Ma Domino receives full information on Darma's history, which then enables her to appreciate its impact and assist Darma's recovery.

How to use this story

- Read the story and talk about how Darma came to Ma Domino's care.

- Social workers may use the story to prepare children for life-story work.

- Explore how the child's strategies enabled their survival in the past but can often be counter-productive in their foster/adoptive/kinship family.

- Through drama, explore how the perceptions of adults and pre-teen children are likely to differ.

- Encourage the children to express their wishes and dreams

Story 3: Darma's despair

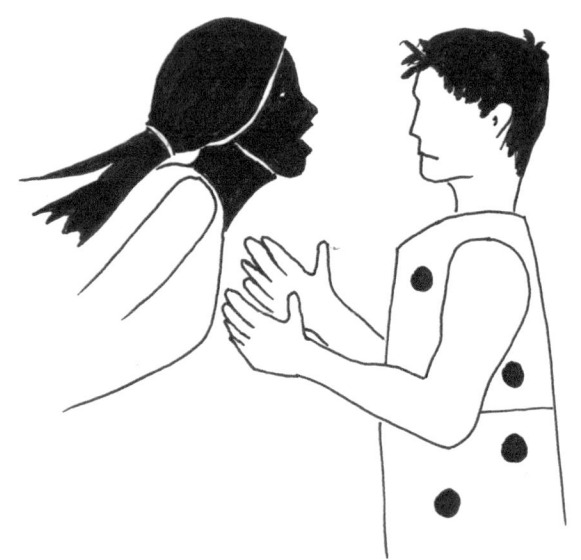

Darma, 14, had been at Ma Dominos since she was 4 years old, when she arrived bent and battered. Memories of her Mum getting horribly damaged by men assaulting her gave Darma nightmares. It had made life so very scary for her that she kept expecting the worst to happen. When anyone tried to be nice to Darma she was on her guard expecting "payback" sooner or later. Ma Domino was kind and gentle so Darma began to relax at home. But at school or when anyone new came to the household, she felt terribly stressed.

Some of Darma's problems came from being neglected when she was little. For example, she had never been taught to tell the time from looking at the clock. If someone asked her to meet them at say quarter to five Darma wasn't sure if it meant before or after five or how long a quarter of an hour was. This meant she was often late or didn't turn up to get the help she needed. Even when her peers were genuinely trying to help her, Darma often sensed they were sneering at her and she was never sure if she could trust anyone. Sometimes when her usual teacher was off, replacement teachers told Darma off in front of the class. It made her feel very embarrassed and humiliated.

Around this time Ma Domino's brother, Dave, was waiting for his new house to be built so moved in with them and took over as a father figure. Having been in the army Dave expected to be obeyed and treated with respect. Darma soon resented being told to stop doing things she was enjoying and get on with her homework. It didn't help that she was usually unsure of what exactly the homework task was. The more Dave pressed Darma the more she shouted back until it came to blows. Both got very wound up and neither could bear to lose face and back down. The slanging matches turned into physical fights. Once it started neither would hear Ma Domino telling them to stop. Darma felt unwanted, stupid, and powerless, like life was out of her control. Desperately unhappy she began to cut her wrists and write suicide notes on the walls. Ma Domino was in despair. She knew Darma was vulnerable but also knew Dave was expecting her to back his authority too. She wondered if she'd been wise to let him stay but he had nowhere else to go and at least he played football and card games with the boys. Ma Domino asked for information about Darma's background. Reading it helped her understand why Darma was so resistant to homework and reactive to people she felt were putting her down.

Ma Domino asked her niece, Dorrie, to help Darma learn about her life story so she'd realise how incredibly brave she'd been in surviving so much terror in her young life. As she acted scenes from her early life, Darma started to appreciate how difficult things had been for her birth parents, who had taken drugs and drunk too heavily to block out their painful memories and feelings of inadequacy. Darma began to tell stories and use her artistic skill to draw pictures to illustrate them. Receiving praise for her pictures helped Darma to feel better. When Dave realised the trauma that Darma had been through, he stopped trying to push her around. Instead he helped her with some of her homework and negotiated time limits for when she would do as he asked. Feeling supported, Darma became more confident about going to school.

Activities

- On a large piece of paper, draw a clock face. Illustrate the sections between each hour with activities that occur during the school day. Draw the Domino characters doing these activities.

- On a second piece of paper, draw a circle to represent one hour. Divide the hour into four quarters to illustrate activities that fill three of the quarter-hours. Divide the fourth quarter into 5 and 10-minute sections. Illustrate activities that fit into these time slots.

- Create your own story and illustrate it. Think of who might help the hero to overcome obstacles and achieve their goal.

- Invite young people to create a collage "all about me" with pictures of their interests, pets, places they like to go or hope to visit, plus photos of themselves, friends and family, sports interests, ambitions etc.

Materials

A1 or A2 sized paper, colour felt tips, pencils, pictures (e.g. from clip art), paint or crayons, photos, collage materials such as glue, glitter and sequins.

Discussion

- How does it feel for a child who can't keep up with her classmates, e.g. due to being unable to tell the time or to understand particular tasks? Why do you think Darma was so anxious in school?

- Can you guess what scary things happened to Darma before she came to Ma Domino's? What worries her now? Do you have these worries?

- What effect did Dave's stay at Ma Domino's have on Darma? Dave and Darma rattled each other. Who would you blame most?

- What do you think was annoying Darma? What makes you anxious? What else might children in new families find hard?

- What encouraged Darma to go to school? How did Ma Domino help? How do you think understanding her life story helped Darma?

- What stories do you like? Shall we write the next chapter to this story?

Reflections

- Darma hated being confronted when she felt unsure of what was being expected of her.

- School made Darma anxious because she found it hard to understand or remember things. Not having learned to tell the time was especially embarrassing for her.

- Severe neglect caused connections to be missing in Darma's brain. This made it difficult for her to remember things people tried to teach her.

- Before she came to Ma Domino's, Darma saw men attacking her Mum. Given sleeping pills by one of her Mum's partners meant her Mum could earn money on the streets and give him the money she earned.

- Due to early trauma, Darma was always scared of strange men. When Dave tried to make her do homework, two traumatic triggers coincided for Darma, sending her anxiety very high. Army life had made Dave intolerant of not having his orders obeyed, which didn't help matters.

- Darma's worst fear about losing her temper and lashing out was that she would never be in control of herself and might kill someone.

- As a person of colour, Darma suffered racist comments about her appearance, particularly her hair.

- Providing the opportunity for Darma to practise tasks she struggled with and encouraging a peer friendship helped her gain the confidence to keep trying. Charts of illustrated clocks helped her learn to tell the time.

- Ma Domino enabled Darma to process her life story and to see herself as a hero.

Sibling rivalry and co-dependence

From an early age, sibling relationships influence the way children make relationships for the rest of their lives. Sibling relationships are often the only ones that span a lifetime, usually lasting long after parents have died. Since children want to please their parents and feel loved and approved of, rivalry almost invariably stems from the fear that a sibling is preferred, loved or admired more than them. Of course age and stage of development requires that children will have different bedtimes, curfews and so on. Some parents show preference for one sibling to enforce the cooperation of both. Although squabbles are normal and the way we learn to deal with conflicts, rivalry between maltreated siblings sometimes requires a far higher level of parental vigilance, which makes the task of parenting them very challenging. Even so, focusing exclusively on the conflict between siblings can overshadow the very processes that facilitate their relationship. Jones (2015) advises caregivers to pay more attention to children's perspectives. Story 4: "Dorrie Loses Davey" focuses on the impact of loss. The disappearance of Davy led Dorrie to discover how important he was to her and feel relief and joy at his return.

How to use the story

- Read the story to convey that children are entitled to be valued equally.

- Encourage insecure children to ask for the reassurance they need.

- Use the creative activities to enhance children's skills at taking turns.

- Invite the children to reflect on their brothers' or sisters' positive qualities and things they would miss if their rival were no longer there.

Story 4: Dorrie loses Davy

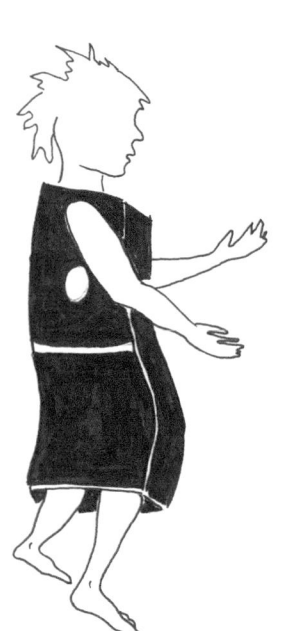

Dorrie, aged 10 and Davy, aged 11, live in a large family of dominoes. As a junior domino, Dorrie wore just one dot. Davy had two dots. He used his extra dot to act superior and would wind Dorrie up by saying irritating things like, "You're only a girl! Boys are far more important!" Dorrie would retort, "Boys are useless, they need girls to look after them." At meal times, these two were squashed up close. Both hated it when the space was so tight, it felt like they could hardly breathe.

One day, Dorrie needed Davy's help. He refused, which made her especially annoyed. Then a row erupted over whose turn it was to start a game. Dorrie kept shouting, "It's my turn!" but Davy went first, yelling, "No, its mine! You went first last time!" No matter how carefully they planned their turns, when it came to it, neither co-operated. This gave Ma Domino a massive headache. "What are we going to do?" she sighed. All of a sudden, Davy skidded off and vanished. "Good!" said Dorrie, feeling very relieved.

Well at first it was peaceful but an hour or so later, when Davy hadn't come back, Dorrie started to feel worried. They searched all over but couldn't find him. Later, as the dominoes slid back into their places, the space left by Davy's absence rattled the rest. Dorrie stood at the door, watching for Davy to reappear. Guessing he'd gone because of her, she felt bad, remembering the many times he'd played with her when no one else had wanted to. As time went on, the rest of them got used to Davy not being there but Dorrie didn't. At times, she thought she saw him but then it turned out to be someone else. Dorrie cried and cried. Even though Davy could be very annoying, she hated him not being around. As she lost interest in playing, her dot faded. Then, one day, a neighbour saw Davy all by himself in a park. Knowing who he was, she took him home. Dorrie was overjoyed to see Davy and he was happy to see her. From then on they decided to keep to the rules they had agreed for sharing. As a result, they didn't fall out quite as often and had loads more fun.

Activities

- Illustrate feelings of emptiness by painting a landscape such as an arctic scene, a desert, a cloudy sky, or an empty beach.

- Think of funny things to say that will help you forget about irritations.

- Working with a partner, take it in turns to pretend to be the foster parent. Bend your foster parent into a shape to express sadness and joy.

- List situations when it can help to have a rota for taking turns.

Materials

Sugar paper, paints and brushes, A4 paper and pens.

Discussion

- Dorrie and Davy often felt "squashed in". Some of us like to sit close to someone and others prefer more room. Who do you like to sit next to?

- Dorrie and Davy squabble as siblings often do. What kind of things do you think they argue about? Do you argue with your brother/sister?

- Do boys need girls more than girls need boys, or just as much? What is the best way to sort out disagreements – shout or talk?

- Have you ever wished for something bad to happen that you later regretted? Most of us say things on impulse, like blaming someone for mistakes we've made. People don't always make it easy for us to put things right.

- How does it feel to lose things? And then to find them?

- How can parents help siblings to get on?

Reflections

- Siblings frequently argue over anything and everything – from who has the most peas on their plate to which is the parent's favourite child.

- Both genders are of equal importance and need each other equally. Charts and timetables help to establish routines and prevent likely disagreements. Talking calmly and not shouting is to be encouraged.

- Sometimes children get scared when their secret wish gets realised. "Magical thinking", which begins around age 3, is the belief that you can make something happen simply by wishing it.

- Losing people you are close to can be very hard. When things go wrong for us, it is tempting to look for someone to blame – even for things we've done ourselves. It helps to learn when to back down from an argument that is difficult to win.

- Talking to a friend helps us cope better with mistakes.

- The value of having a sibling is the prospective companionship of a life-long relationship and their availability to practise dealing with conflict as well as competition.

- Parents/caregivers help by not taking sides with one sibling over another and by encouraging friendships.

Contact with birth family

Children's need for contact and information about their birth family changes as they grow up. An American study by Grotevant et al. (2011) found that contact between adoptive families and their children's birth relatives is beneficial for promoting the young people's adoptive identity. The most influential factor, which Neil (2019) observed to affect outcomes, was new parents' openness to contact. Still, birth parents' mental illness, personality disorder and substance addiction pose risks to the emotional well-being of children in contact with them. As the children approach adolescence, they need to emotionally separate from parents/caregivers in order to move towards independence.

For adopted and fostered children, conflicts can arouse feelings of difference and isolation. The child, who has not understood her birth parent's problems may muse, "If only my real Mum (or Dad) knew where I was she'd come for me and life would be perfect!" Social media has made it far easier for this contact to be made in secret via access to sites such as Whats App, Snapchat and Facebook. Simpson (2013) suggests ways this can be managed. Story 5 is a cautionary tale (based on real-life situations), illustrating what can happen when a young person secretly makes contact with their birth parent. It aims to help young people to recognise the potential dangers. In the story Darcy contacts her birth mother against the advice of her older sister, and is abducted. Even after she has been rescued, regular contact with her birth mother leads Darcy to self-harm and be hospitalised.

How to use the story

- Read the story and ensure your children know where they can access support before they take risks that threaten their future well-being.

- Encourage the child to sever contact with birth parents, who are actively trying to undermine the foster, kinship or adoptive placement.

- Dramatise the story to help your child understand the risks, realise why they were fostered or adopted, be reassured they are wanted and will have many more rewarding experiences in their caregiving family.

Story 5: Darcy's ordeal

Darcy, 13, had been at Ma Dominos since she was 2. Her birth Mum, Baz, contacted her on Facebook. Intrigued, Darcy agreed to a chat in a café near where she lived. One day after school, as Darcy and her boyfriend Alfie went to the place where they'd agreed to meet they saw a car pull up. Baz told Darcy to get in. Alfie, told her not to, but Baz put her hand on Darcy's back and shoved her into the car, saying, "I'm taking you home to live with me!" Baz asked Darcy to sit next to her but Darcy sat by the window. Alfie slid into the seat between Darcy and Baz. In the front, someone Baz said was her sister, sat next to the driver. Darcy hoped to get out when the car stopped at traffic lights but the child locks were on. She felt scared. During the journey she and Alfie text messaged each other and her brother, Dan. Furious, Baz

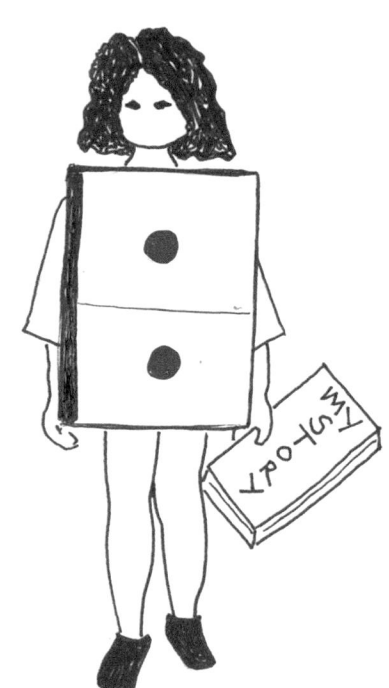

punched Alfie in the face. Darcy texted Dan the name on a signpost she'd seen. Dan told the police. Their texting helped the police to track them.

When they arrived at Baz's house and went in, Baz locked the front door and kept hold of the keys. Wildly hyper, Baz bounced around like a 4-year-old. Her high-pitched voice took Darcy by surprise as she'd always imagined her Mum having a deep voice. Baz asked if they were hungry. Darcy asked if they could go to a restaurant. The aunt said, "That's a nice idea – I'll go and get changed," but Baz said "No!" The walls were covered with pictures of Darcy throughout her childhood, and of Baz's other children. It felt weird especially as Baz had told her she'd never wanted any of her ten kids. She'd loved being pregnant but as soon as the baby was born and people's attention switched away from her to the baby, her interest in the baby waned. Baz made Darcy a cup of tea. After drinking it, Darcy felt tired, sick and kind of weird. Alfie had seen Baz slip a pill in the cup, so he refused a drink. Baz asked Darcy, "Does my baby girl want to lie down?"

Baz kept touching Darcy, fiddling with her hair in a way that made Darcy feel very uncomfortable. Baz told them tales about the past but kept contradicting herself. She said Darcy's adoptive Mum had snatched Darcy from her arms but the details she gave didn't make sense. Later Darcy found out that none of it was true. Baz announced that Darcy's birth Dad, Ben, was coming round. Hearing someone batter at the door, Darcy went into the kitchen, where she lay on the floor, terrified. When it turned out to be the police, she was relieved. Though they had come for Baz, they interviewed Darcy and Alfie and took their phones. While Darcy and Alfie were in the car waiting to be taken home, the police arrested Baz and the other woman, handcuffed them and put them in the other car. As it drove off, Darcy saw Baz give her an evil look that really scared her. In the end, the police charged Baz with injuring Alfie but not for abduction. Darcy and Baz got their phones back a month later.

When they got home, Ma Domino asked for a hug, but Darcy backed off, feeling churned up and confused. Even though Baz had kidnapped and frightened her, she still felt a connection and wanted her approval. Darcy wasn't ready to let go of the fantasy she'd held all through her life – that Baz loved her and if only she knew where Darcy lived, she'd come for her and they'd live happily ever after, like in fairy tales. Dan was jealous that Darcy had got to meet Baz and he hadn't. Darcy had always blamed social workers for not allowing her to FaceTime Baz but found out Ma Domino had refused when asked a year ago. Darcy reckoned that if she'd had contact, none of this would have happened, though knew Ma had just been trying to protect her.

After a few days, Baz sent Darcy a message and they talked via FaceTime. One day, Baz passed the phone to Darcy's Dad, Ben. Darcy said "Hello!" Ben told Baz off for interrupting or saying something horrible. Darcy chatted, having forgotten the accounts of how violent he'd been in the past. Baz kept saying weird stuff. She got very angry and told Darcy she was going to shoot herself. Then Baz disappeared off the screen, giving the impression she was dead. Darcy was terrified but two hours later she saw Baz alive, watching TV. Darcy was so upset she cut her wrists and spent several days in hospital. When doctors said she was ok to go home, she didn't want to leave, scared Baz would be waiting for her. Darcy stopped making FaceTime contact with Baz and Ben. Her life became a bit calmer. Even so, Darcy kept worrying about what she'd do if Baz ever showed up. Ma Domino helped her work out which people she could phone and the places she could go, to keep herself safe.

Activities

- With your adoptive/foster family, dramatise a scene from the story or make up your own version. Decide what happens next.

- Draw Baz as a domino. Is she smooth or sharp? Battered or sleek?

- Make a list of people you could go to if you needed someone to talk to.

- Create a montage of pictures of yourself and your family.

Materials

Card, paper, scissors, photos, glue stick, felt tips.

Discussion

- Was it a good idea for Darcy to make contact with her birth parents without telling Ma Domino? Where may be a safe place to meet them?

- Alfie came too. How might this have affected him? What risks did Darcy take by letting him come with her? How scary is it to be locked up?

- How did Darcy know that Baz was lying to her about her adoptive parents? How can you tell when people are being truthful or not?

- Darcy dreamed of her adoptive mother finding her. Do you have these dreams? Can you tell me about them or paint a picture?

- It was a big shock when Baz tricked Darcy by making her think she'd died. Has anyone tricked you? How do you keep safe on social media?

- What advice would you give friends who wanted to trace their birth family and meet them, not knowing everything about them?

Reflections

- Before children make contact with birth parents on social media, they should always tell their adoptive/foster parents. There may be no safe way to meet mentally ill birth parents. If the child arranges to meet them, it needs to be in a public place, with a friend or caregiving parent present, in case there are problems such as described in the story.

- For Alfie, the journey to Darcy's birth Mum's house would also have been traumatic as he was potentially as much at risk as Darcy. There could have been an accident. The birth parent's partner might have a violent temper. Alfie's text message to Darcy's brother helped the police to track the phone and rescue them.

- Baz locked them in because she didn't want to risk them escaping. Darcy knew Baz's account of adopters snatching her was a lie as she'd seen photos of the handover and heard her adoptive Mum's account. Some lie so convincingly it's not always easy to detect this.

- The police should have charged Baz with kidnapping or abduction but the ages of the children made the police unsure of a conviction.

- Adopted children often have idyllic dreams of being rescued by birth parents and are deeply shocked when they find out the real truth.

- It is important for children to delete contacts with people who threaten their safety. The best advice is to get all the information about the child's history before the child commits to meeting birth parents, whose particular difficulties may stop them from being able to provide the quality of relationship the child hopes for.

Social isolation

In the light of the Coronavirus pandemic, the threats of similar viruses and the uncertainty as to when "normal life" will resume, here I reflect on the impact of enforced social isolation for adoptive, foster and kinship families. In the UK, the requirement to stay at home that began on 24 March 2020 led to all schools, colleges, leisure, entertainment and sports facilities closing. Shops selling non-essential items followed. Roads and parks soon emptied. As we learned to social distance ourselves, a new way of being began. Noting that our world became a new world, Holmwood (2021) observes the reality of the pandemic made it hard for us to distance ourselves as we would in a hypothetical drama. After all this was real life theatre from which we could not escape, its heightened reality promulgated by the regular broadcasts on television on rising numbers of deaths and shortages of protective equipment.

Meanwhile having to stay at home has restricted many from being able to "do" anything other than just "be". The state of "not knowing" when lockdown will end has left families powerless to make plans and many to be financially impacted. Parents struggled to reassure children, who having already lost important attachment relationships, dreaded abandonment. The fear of death raises immense anxiety especially when the caregiving parents get sick.

Parents have had to extend their roles to include teaching, as well as giving their children emotional support. Some families are being therapeutically and/or educationally supported by phone and video link. This has its limitations but many find it better than no support. Stories and story-making are effective for stimulating imagination and providing a structure that enables feelings and experience to be processed so that new understandings can be reached. For these children, a benefit of being at home is the gift of time to receive precious parental attention, compensating for deficits in their past.

How to use this story

- Read Story 6 and draw from the discussion points.

- Encourage children to get fresh air and try out the creative activities.

Story 6: Disruption for Derry

Derry, now 12, was five days old when social workers took him to foster care. This was because his birth father had an alcohol problem and his birth Mum was mentally unwell. By the time Derry was 7, his foster father, Dennis was drinking heavily. His foster Mum, Dolores, was so afraid she left but he didn't let her take Derry. One day Dennis passed out drunk on the sofa. Derry knocked at the neighbours' door to ask for food. They called the police and Derry got taken to Ma Domino's. Derry was then able to see Dolores (who in his eyes was his real Mum) but struggled with schoolwork and got bullied. Ma Domino was kind and helped him with homework so things got better.

One day everything changed when a virus spread like wildfire not just round Planet Domino but right across the stratosphere! The school closing was quite a relief for Derry. What really bothered him was not being able to see his best mate and worse still, being prevented from visiting Dolores. Derry couldn't phone her because she didn't have a smart phone with which she could talk to him so he worried about her. He'd seen the man she was living with just once but it was enough to know he didn't like or trust him. Derry was scared this man would keep her prisoner using lockdown as an excuse to control her.

At Ma Domino's it was more crowded than usual because no one was getting out to school or socialising. Tempers flared. There didn't seem to be any way of settling squabbles since everyone was scared to go outside in case they caught the virus. Some of the older ones were very stressed about whether their girlfriend or boyfriend was breaking up with them. Derry started writing a list of everyone he knew. He put the names into two columns according to whom he thought was most likely to die and who might live. Another person had been sent to stay at Ma Domino's. As a result, Derry had to share a room with Dudley, which meant far less privacy. His birthday was coming soon and Dudley was scared that if his party didn't happen he wouldn't grow any older. He started having accidents that left the bathroom and sometimes, their bedroom, very smelly. All these things gave Derry a massive headache.

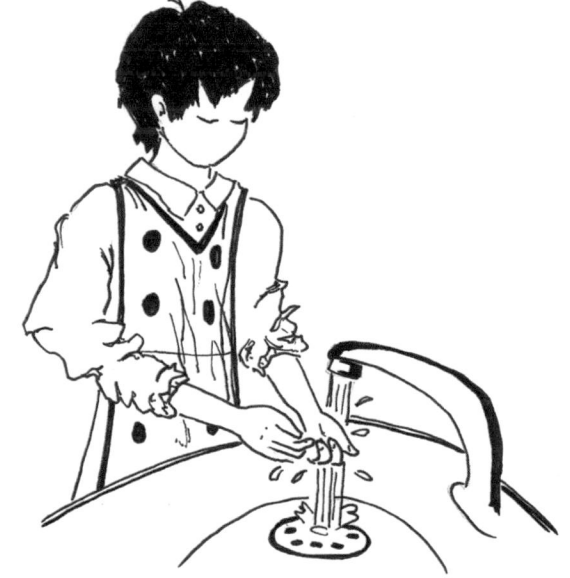

Because of the virus they all had to wash their hands frequently. As Derry's anxiety got worse he was longer washing his hands, not just every time there was a reason to, but frequently in between. Derry wasn't sleeping well because he was worrying about Dolores, about himself dying from the virus, and about Dudley and others at Ma Domino's, who had problems – in fact he had nightmares. When Ma Domino realised how worried Derry was about Dolores she phoned the domestic violence unit at Domino Police Station. They knew Dolores and promised regular checks on her. Derry was very relieved to hear this. He and Ma Domino talked about the pressures they were all under and agreed that creating routines, rituals and lists of things to do would help.

Activities

- Go out for a walk, run, bike ride or practise hitting a ball against a wall.

- Find out if volunteers are needed for jobs you can do to help others.

- Do exercise videos that are fun to move around or dance to.

- Make a list of films to watch and work out a timetable for them.

- Tidy and organise your room, clothes and equipment.

- Have a storytelling hour to share the best stories and books.

- Play cards and board games you haven't played for ages.

- Dig out jigsaws and work out which ones are complete.

- Listen to your favourite music compilations.

- Arrange a virtual party with your friends and play charades.

- Bake biscuits or make pizzas with toppings showing expressions.

- Take a virtual field trip round famous places.

- Paint pictures, using images available on the computer.

- Design a room to decorate when the shut-down ends.

- Interview each other about how social isolation affects you.

Materials

Bats and balls, bikes, exercise videos, books, cards, board games, jigsaws, laptop, cooking ingredients, paint and brushes, paper

Discussion

- What is it like to be in foster care?

- How do you think Derry's birth family history affected him?

- Why do you think he regarded his foster Mum as his "real" Mum?

- Why did Derry worry about her?

- I wonder how she came to be with another controlling partner?

- What might it be like to have your foster parent get very drunk?

- How do you think it felt for Derry to be behind the others in his class?

- Do you find homework difficult?

- How do you avoid bullies?

- How has the lockdown affected you?

- Are you able to get outside?

- Is there somewhere you can go safely if you want to be on your own?

- What things have restricted you most?

- What do you miss the most?

- Have other young people's worries affected you? Which ones?

- What worries you the most? Are there any ways I can help?

- How do you work out sharing the space?

- How do you agree on respecting each other's privacy?

- What is your favourite music or activity?

- How would you like the story to turn out?

Reflections

- Some children in foster, adoptive or kinship care feel stigmatised for not being in their birth family. Even young people, who are relieved to be safe, are likely to have worries, perhaps about bullying, what will happen to them next, how much choice they will have over their future, how they will keep up with their friends and so on.

- For Derry, being removed from his birth parents at five days old would likely have left him feeling disconnected, anxious about where he belongs. A further move added to his sense of abandonment.

- Derry didn't remember his birth Mum, only his foster Mum, so he saw her as his "real" Mum because she looked after him. He worried about her making poor choices. Derry didn't trust her latest partner. His foster father had also been a drinker, unsupportive and very controlling. Having a foster parent get drunk would add to a child's sense of abandonment and left Derry feeling unsafe and frightened.

- It is embarrassing for children to lag way behind their peers and may incline them to give up trying. Homework can be difficult if you don't fully understand what is expected of you. Derry would try to avoid bullies by keeping out of their way and making sure that an adult was near enough to help him, if he felt scared.

- Lockdown has been beneficial for some children in releasing them from the pressures of normal life. But many miss their friends and worry that if they are not quick enough in responding to text messages, they will be excluded from their friendship group. Some children are not getting out for exercise and fresh air, which are essential for healthy development.

- Probably the most frustrating aspect was the impossibility of being able to plan ahead and know when it was going to be lifted safely.

2 Trauma, abuse and neglect

Trauma

The experience of subjection to neglect, domestic violence and parents' substance misuse is extremely traumatic for children. Polyvagal Theory (Porges and Daniel, 2017) explains why physical sensation is even more immediate than the psychological. The child, who is hyper-aroused, will be unable to concentrate on anything else, due to a sense of being unsafe. Abused children often hate themselves and fear getting things wrong. Many shut down their feelings but sensory triggers of certain sights, sounds, smells and textures reignite their brain's alarm system (the amygdala) that triggers fight-flight-freeze reactions. Experiencing the (past) traumatic event as recurring in the present moment places the child in a state of abject terror and emotional paralysis.

When the healthy brain is faced with something threatening, it accesses the "reasoning" hippocampus, which checks with the higher cortex to weigh up the scale of the threat – "Was that a gunshot or something falling off a shelf?" This checking process takes about seven seconds, to decide what to do. But when threats keep repeating, excessive quantities of the neurochemical, cortisol, destroy these connections. The reasoning part of the brain shuts down so the brain relies on lower parts warning, "This has happened before!" The child won't remember the trauma and fearing annihilation, is unable to explain his reaction. Specialist assessment may be needed to help him.

One way to help trauma-triggered children to cope better is to encourage them to notice the physical effects on them. We can invite the child to recall their bodily sensations, such as feeling hot, having sweaty palms, stomach churning or their legs feeling the urge to run. This awareness can buy them time to find a safe place or to tell someone who understands. Most important is to help the child feel safe. The benefit of stories is that their fictional context allows privacy and distance for talking about feelings that are real.

Verbal abuse and neglect

Being on the receiving end of verbal abuse, persistent denigration and insults cause even more lasting damage to the child's developing brain than physical abuse, according to Teicher et al. (2016), albeit frequently combined with other forms of abuse such as chronic neglect and being witness to incidents of domestic violence and parents' substance misuse. Degli-Esposti et al. (2019) find neglect continuing to be the most common reason for children being subject of child protection. The traumatic impact of neglect came to attention with the publication of research on brain scans of Romanian institution children, deprived of touch and toys, and often diseased. Their brains had entire black holes in place of connected neurons in the orbito-frontal cortex (Gerhardt, 2004). Recent research (Mackes et al., 2020) finds these children's brains to be 8.6% smaller than those of other adoptees. Abuse, intentional or not, affects all brain parts and has long-term effects.

Story 7 "Dudley who thought he was Dud" describes the distressing impact of verbal abuse, which leaves a child feeling worthless. The story conveys that helping someone else can bring desired friendship and acceptance.

How to use this story

- Read the story. Scenes from it can be dramatised between two people (parent and child) or in small groups of children as a means of enabling them to practise at friendship skills, show interest in other people and offer help when opportunities arise.

- Help the child to think of other ways that Dudley could have pulled himself out of his difficult situation.

- Encourage traumatised children to recognise their bodily sensations while they are acting in a fictional role. For example in a scene between King and servant, does the King's face go red when he's cross? This will give the child privacy to learn about feelings (as the feeling is attached to the role). Noticing how these sensations affect children in real-life situations when they are feeling angry, scared, upset, can buy them time to tell someone who understands or to find somewhere they feel safe.

- If the traumatised child continues to be upset and unable to manage their feelings to the extent that they are hurting themselves and others, you may need to arrange a specialist assessment to ensure that their needs are met appropriately.

Story 7: Dudley, who thought he was Dud.

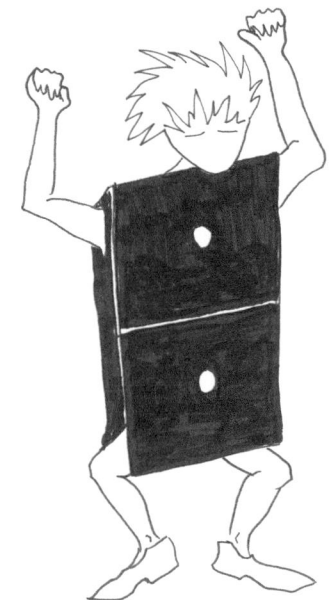

Dudley was the youngest of a large family, who called him "Dud". His birth parents didn't look after their children at all well. They just bickered and fought all the time. There was never enough food to go round and Dud's tummy often ached with hunger. When the electric meter was empty, draughts whistled through the house. Doors slid off their hinges and things got battered and fell apart. So the family kept moving house and more people joined it or left. This happened so often that Dud got very confused. You see, as so many adults came and left the family, he wasn't even certain which of them were his Mum and Dad. His brothers and sisters kept saying, "Dud, you're an idiot!" They showed their sharp edges, setting him up to get blamed when things went missing or got broken. Dud felt stupid and unwanted. One day, he got thrown out like a piece of trash.

Dud was 10 when he was taken to a new family where the mother, Ma Domino, was warm and welcoming. But to Dud it felt weird. Everything smelled and tasted strange. There were lots more names to learn, which didn't help. A domino called Dom asked Dud his name. He replied, "Dud". The others laughed. Ma Domino said, "His name is Dudley! He's been called Dud for short." Then she asked Dud, "What would you like us to call you?" Dud shrugged, not knowing what to say. Ma suggested "Let's call you Dudley. It's your real name and its much nicer." Dudley had to go to a new school, which meant new routines, new names, new buildings, as well as learning new rules. He dreaded making mistakes but couldn't help it because he'd missed a lot of school. Dudley often gave the wrong answer and Dom, who was in the same class, yelled, "Its Dudley the Dud!" This reminded Dudley of how bad his family had always made him feel. Upset and furious, he thumped Dom, not knowing how else to shut him up. The teacher was cross with them both and told Ma Domino about it.

One day, Dom kicked his ball over the wall into a garden next to their school. Dom didn't want to lose the ball but knew he'd be in big trouble if he tried to retrieve it. Dudley said, "I'll get it!" He climbed over the wall, picked up the ball and tossed it over. Luckily, no one else saw him and Dom was very grateful. After that, Dom saw Dudley as a mate worth having and stuck up for him. They became friends and enjoyed sharing games and going to the park together. If anyone needed help with a tricky situation, Dom told the person to ask Dudley. That helped him make even more friends. Soon Dudley stopped worrying so much. He managed to concentrate better and learn faster.

Activities

- In pairs, talk about what calms you down when you feel anxious.

- In small groups or pairs act out a scene from the story, from the point of view of the teacher, Dom, Ma Domino, or one of the other students.

- Make clay models of Dudley's birth family. Notice how fragile they are. Then remake them as sturdier versions of Ma Domino's family. Later, you can paint the models and use them to create another story.

Materials

Air-drying clay and tools for shaping, e.g. kitchen knife, spoon, fork.

Discussion

- When changes happen too fast, it is hard to remember everything. How have you found changes in your life?

- Dudley's family called him "Dud". What is it like to be called names?

- Ma Domino proposed to drop the nickname "Dud". Did that help?

- Do you find it hard to answer grownups' questions sometimes?

- Dudley hated making mistakes. What encourages you to keep trying?

- Can you think of other ways to help children feel included in a group?

- Was Dudley wrong to trespass in order to get Dom's ball back?

- Can you think of other ways Dudley could have helped Dom?

Reflections

- Difficult changes that children undergo include moving in with a new family, adjusting to new siblings, relatives, new house, neighbourhood, school and the contact arrangements with the child's birth family.

- Being called nasty, derogatory names damages the child's brain. It causes low self-esteem and anxiety and affects the child's learning.

- It is possible Dudley might have been too embarrassed to answer Ma Domino straight away, or he may have been so used to being put down that he hadn't thought to question being called "Dud".

- Having a grownup listen carefully and making a friend of his own age encouraged Dudley to keep trying even when he made mistakes.

- To help children feel included you could invite them to join in a game, activity or outing. Teachers can arrange the classroom so that the child can sit in a small group.

- It is wrong and illegal to trespass on another's property but in this story, no harm was done. In collecting the ball, Dudley helped Dom and won his admiration and respect. Children can be encouraged to think of other ways for Dom to make friends.

- Dom should really have told a teacher and arranged to call at the house to ask the owner to return the ball to him.

Sexual abuse

Sexual abuse is damaging to the child's developing brain (Teicher et al., 2016; Van der Kolk, 2005). It is an abuse of power from which young children cannot protect themselves. Sexual abuse frequently occurs within the family. The vast majority (though not all) of perpetrators are male adults. Fear of the abuser may deter the non-abusing parent from protecting their children. The children will not know that what is being done to them is abnormal until they find out (usually at school) that it doesn't happen to all children. Childhood Sexual Abuse includes Child Sexual Exploitation (Kelly and Karsna, 2018) in recognition that the capacity to give informed consent to sex is manipulated and undermined. Abuse makes it difficult for the recipients to form trustworthy relationships. An example of their vulnerability is the abused 11-year-old, who asks people she hardly knows, things like, "Do you think I'm sexy?"

The abused child learns to develop strategies of coercion, defensiveness and helplessness as their means of survival. For instance, getting physically close with someone may encourage that person to be kind and feed the child. Strategies become fixed unless or until the victims gain emotional security.

Story 8 "Dotty tries to dominate", describes the damaging effects of betrayal on an abused child whose mother failed to protect her even when begged to. Years later, Dotty seeks excitement and is afraid to display any weakness in case it leads to rejection. A new friendship and activity help her to adjust.

How to use this story

- Read Story 8. Help the children to think of dangerous situations. Explain their rights to privacy and protection.

- Encourage the children to practise ways of saying "no" to unwelcome invitations and taking charge of their body's safety.

- Helplines such as Childline give advice to children who feel too scared to tell the people they know.

- Ask the child/ren what help Dotty needs. What advice would they give a friend who was being dared to do something they know is too risky.

- Explore why the mother in the story was too scared to protect Dotty.

- Point out that no adult should try to hurt and frighten children.

- If children disclose sexual abuse, even if this abuse occurred in the past, it needs to be reported, following the local safeguarding procedures, to ensure the protection of that child and other children.

- Some children will also be entitled to financial compensation.

Story 8: Dotty tries to dominate

Dotty, aged 12, was in Dolly's class at school. Sometimes they hung out together because they were both mates with Dina, although they didn't always get on.

Dotty was living at Ma Domino's because she was unsafe in her birth family. Her Dad used to play games that made her feel yucky, sticky and scared. Dotty had shouted for help but Mum never came to stop him because she too was scared. Dad was often in a bad mood and hiding from the authorities.

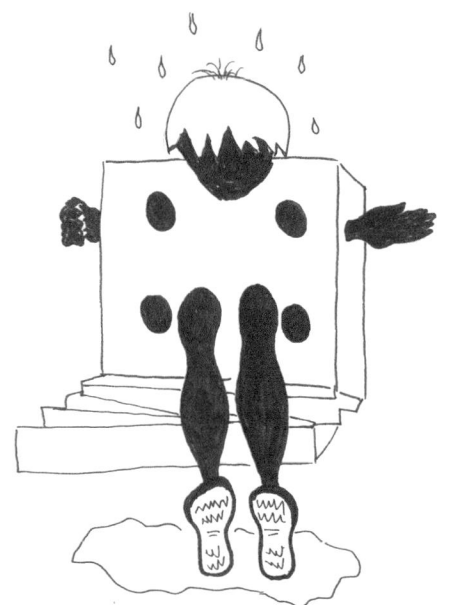

Dotty used to ask Mum what she was thinking about but Mum's face was like a mask, closed up and unreadable. To Dotty, it felt like being locked out in the rain, abandoned. Everything seemed random, like no one had ever "joined the dots" and explained things in ways she could understand. Even now Dotty struggled to make sense of why people did the things they did or to know what might happen next. She had to guess so she made up her own rules as she went along but often felt horribly left out.

At school, Dotty noticed that people were avoiding her. She sensed they didn't like or trust her. She embellished the stories she told to win attention, but most people didn't believe her. It made her want to scream. What Dotty hated most of all was being ignored – that felt like having a knife plunged into an open cut. When things were quiet, Dotty tried to liven them up. "Join my gang!" she'd say to her classmates, who found it hard to say "no" to her. One day, she dared Dolly and Dina to climb over a toilet partition onto an unsuspecting victim in the next cubicle. Dina refused but Dolly did it to impress Dotty. Of course, the victim was very upset and told her parents. Then they told the Head, who asked Ma Domino to come to a meeting to discuss it.

At the end of the school day Ma Domino saw Dolly at the school gate and asked her why she stayed friends with Dotty since it was causing massive problems. Dolly explained, "Dotty hasn't got any friends except Dina and me and I don't want to break up with Dina." Then Dotty came out of the classroom and Ma Domino asked "Shall we invite Dolly home for tea? We can find an activity you'll both enjoy, then we'll get everyone together to talk about how to deal with these situations that I'm getting called in to school about."

The next day Dolly came round after school, Ma Domino had a large box of beads of varying shape and colours, ready to thread. "Choose the beads you like", she said and suggested they make friendship bracelets. Dotty found the bracelet making easier than she'd expected and really enjoyed herself.

Ma Domino reminded them that if they ever felt bored or anxious, they could fiddle with these beads, to remind themselves of their friendships. Then they could make plans to have some fun and feel better about things. While the girls ate their meal, they chatted with the others about school, who they got on with and why. It led to talking about ways to avoid fights with bullies.

From then on, Dotty kept the bracelet with her. She and Dolly stayed friends, and helped each other to stay out of trouble, at least, for some of the time.

Activities

- In small groups, make bracelets using a selection of beads. Choose beads that remind you of your best memories.

- In groups, write a play about friendship and how to nurture it. Talk about what friends are for and how you support each other.

- In pairs make a collage of images of your friends and shared interests.

- Make plans to meet and try out a new interest such as a dance class.

Materials

Beads, thread, fastenings, collage materials, paper, pens, scissors and card.

Discussion

- Dotty had frightening memories of her time in her birth family. Do you think her Dad might never have felt safe when he was a child?

- I wonder if Dotty's Mum was too scared of Dotty's Dad to protect her. How does it feel to try talking to someone whose face is closed up?

- Can you tell if someone is acting in an unsafe way? Are there signs like being asked to keep nasty secrets or having your friendships restricted?

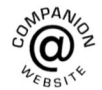

- Can you think of ways that children can protect themselves from unsafe adults? Who should they confide in? Do you know of any telephone helplines for children? Shall we write down the number?

- How might it feel to be abandoned and sense that you don't belong?
  Dotty struggled to recognise or understand other people's feelings. How could you help someone like her to make a friend?

- It is very upsetting to be ignored while others are getting the attention and things you want or need. What helps you feel more valued?

- What advice would you give a friend who has been dared to do something stupid? How could a parent or teacher or classmate help Dotty?

- Ma Domino involved the girls in making jewellery. How did it help?

Reflections

- We can guess that Dotty's Dad abused her when she lived with him.

- Dotty's Mum would probably have been too scared to confront him.

- The closed face and lack of response from Dotty's mum would have left Dotty feeling very left out, rejected, as if she didn't matter.

- When someone asks a child to keep worrying secrets, or tries to control their friendships and other aspects of their life, it is a warning sign that such a person is not safe to be with.

- If a child feels unsafe, they need to find an adult who will believe them – perhaps a teacher, counsellor, social worker, police officer or Childline.

- The feeling of being abandoned and not belonging can leave a child alienated and unhappy. It can wreck their peace of mind and ability to concentrate.

- Inviting Dotty to play a game at lunchtime could help her feel welcome.

- A friend dared to do something likely to get them into trouble can be encouraged to talk about it to someone they trust to give wise advice.

- Enabling a child like Dotty to join in social activities may help.

- Teachers can try to encourage children. Foster/adoptive parents can provide funds and transport needed to engage in social activities.

- Being invited to make jewellery helped Dotty to forge a friendship and stay out of trouble.

Memory problems

The parts of the brain that are used to recall the past are the same as those used to imagine the future and are usually well honed by age 9. Perry and Szalavitz (2017; 2008) warn that these parts fail to develop if not stimulated. The connections in neglected children's brains can be uneven, which results in variation in ability across subject areas. Consequently, teachers assume that the child is not trying hard enough at the tasks they genuinely struggle with. Patchy neural development makes it difficult for the child to anticipate and plan ahead. Criticism discourages and inclines the child to give up.

Story 9 "Dom the Domino" demonstrates the "domino effect" whereby one decision affects another, which then affects the next and so on. The story suggests ways of helping children who have memory problems to recognise consequences, avert disaster and feel motivated to improve their coping skills.

How to use this story

- Parents, teaching staff, social workers or counsellors can read Story 9 to illustrate the consequences of actions and explain the advantages for children to train themselves to put systems in place, then follow these systems and hopefully, enjoy more reciprocal relationships.

- Use Worksheet 1 to encourage the children to think of helpful routines and memory aids, e.g. for organising their clothes and equipment.

- Explore the benefits of homework and school projects and for the child, of asking for the help they need.

Story 9: Dom the Domino

"Dom", short for "Dominic" is 10 and lives in Ma Domino's large family. Ma Domino had fostered him since he was a baby, when his Mum had given him away. One night, Dom was up playing long past his usual bedtime. The next day, he was late getting up for school. Ma Domino kept calling. "Get a move on! If you don't get up, you'll be late, and that means you'll be in trouble! Come on, Dom, your brother's downstairs, he's ready and waiting for you!" Dom felt tired and edgy as he searched for his school uniform. He yelled, "Where are my dots?" Ma Domino replied,

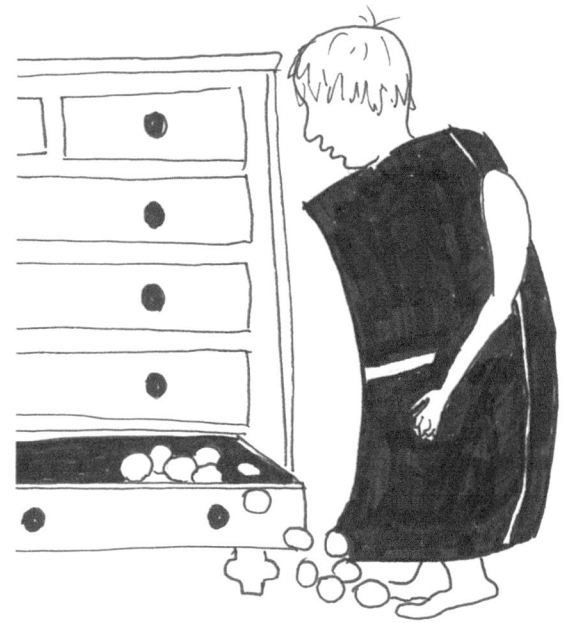

"They'll be where you left them!" As he reached into his drawer, loads of them spilled out on to the floor. Dom piled the dots into a heap, moaning, "Now I'll be really late!" Already, things were stacking up against him and the day had hardly started! On the way to school, his brother, Davy, started making domineering remarks so Dom tripped him up. Davy fell in a puddle, pulling Dom on top of him so now they were muddy as well as late!

At school they joined the queue lining up to go in. Dom remembered he'd left his packed lunch behind. Cursing, he fell against his brother and, yes, you've guessed it! The whole group toppled over. The teacher yelled, "I saw that! Go to the Head Teacher's office – you're getting a detention!" Dom insisted he didn't mean to push anyone. The Head didn't believe him and told him off for lying. From then on, Dom's day got worse and worse! By the afternoon, he was hungry, tired and fed up. The teacher phoned Ma Domino to tell her that Dom would be late home after detention. Ma said, "but he'll be starving! I've found his lunchbox." She explained, "he didn't sleep at all well last night!"

The teacher said "Ok, I'll let him off this time so long as you tell him what the consequences will be if it happens again!" Ma Domino promised she would. Later, she helped Dom think of ways he could make his life go more smoothly. Dom knew she wanted him to get more sleep, do his homework, and keep his dots tidy. He promised to try not to annoy the teacher in future.

Activities

- In pairs, create a domino run. As the adult retells the story the child or children set up a domino for each decision that Dom made.

- Notice how much harder things got for Dom.

- Think of five advantages to being organised and five ways to achieve it.

- In small groups, using Worksheet 1, list ways to make your life easier – such as keeping clothes and equipment tidy – then decorate the chart.

Materials

Sets of dominoes, card and felt tips.

Discussion

- Dom had a bad day at school. How does a bad day feel for you?

- Going to bed late made him tired in the morning. What time do you go to bed? How many hours of sleep do you think you need at your age?

- Would keeping your things tidy save you time?

- What did Dom forget to take to school? What happened as a result? How did Davy get on Dom's nerves? What might help them get on?

- Was it fair of the teacher to give Dom a detention? Is it right for all children to be treated the same? Why or why not?

- How did Ma Domino help? If you are having a bad day, do you have someone you can talk to? Who can you go to for help or advice?

- How might Dom get on for the rest of that week?

- What would help you most if you were in Dom's situation?

Reflections

- A bad day makes you feel miserable and expect nothing to go right. In general, children aged 10 will benefit from being in bed by 9 p.m. and at age 14, by 10 p.m., so that they get enough sleep.

- Keeping things tidy and knowing where to find them saves a lot of time.

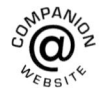

- Forgetting his lunchbox put Dom in a bad mood as he realised he'd be hungry. Davy would have made him feel irritable and silly. Dom could apologise and make it up with Davy, say, by inviting him to play a game.

- One rule for everyone is usually fair and easy for the class to understand. But the "one-size-fits-all" approach doesn't always help children who have special needs. Fortunately the teacher relented when Ma Domino explained why Dom was having problems.

- Sometimes parents have to argue for their child and ask teachers to be flexible so that their child's special needs can be met.

- It can be helpful for children to have a named person they can go to in times of need. It is important for them to have someone they can talk to when they are struggling, who can advocate on their behalf if needed.

Foetal alcohol spectrum

Foetal alcohol spectrum disorder (FASD) is a condition that is caused during pregnancy by the mother's long-term use of alcohol (Lu and Johnson, 2019). It delays brain development but the extent of a child's difficulties in processing data and gaining social understanding may only become apparent at around age 10, when they are expected to be able to work more independently. Children with FASD struggle to recognise social signals or act as expected of their age. They need help with schoolwork and relationships but their disability is invisible so expectations of them are often unrealistic. The repercussions of not having support lead all too frequently to teenage pregnancy and crime.

Illustrating the effects of FASD, Story 10, "Ditty's delight", is about a child, who breaches the social rules she has not learned. Ditty "takes without asking" – a phrase used to describe theft in a literal way – until having her sensory needs met helps her to feel safer, practise better self-control and make friends.

How to use this story

- Read the story. Use the creative and sensory activities to enable the affected child to learn and understand social rules and expectations.

- Use visual formats such as films, cartoons, and dramatic play to help children with FASD learn non-verbal signals and communication skills.

- Provide sensory materials for (safe) touching.

- Get specialist assessment to ensure the child's needs are met.

- Before allowing lotion sharing, ensure that children, who may have been abused, don't find this threatening or uncomfortable.

Story 10: Ditty's delight

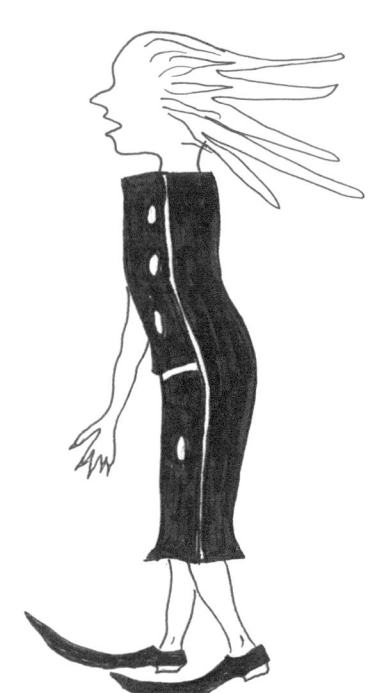

Ditty Domino, aged 10, couldn't keep still. She did things that made her classmates scared of her. If she wanted something belonging to another child, she'd scratch the child with her sharp nails until they handed it over! Having their treasures made Ditty feel better and made sure that people noticed her but her classmates were fed up with her and tried to keep out of her way.

Ditty had recently started at the school, having been taken to Ma Domino's because her last foster parents decided they couldn't cope with her. Ditty never gave a reason for doing things that upset other people. Worried, her teacher phoned Ma Domino, explaining, "I'm sure Ditty wants friends but she really isn't helping herself!" Ma Domino replied, "Perhaps she's feeling lost and hurt." An idea suddenly came to her. "I'll bring some hand lotion for Ditty to have at break. It will soften her sharp nails and the smell might remind her not to scratch the other children."

That evening after school, Ma Domino put a tube of hand lotion in Ditty's school bag and gave Ditty a pretty pink drawing book, explaining, "I know you want friends and I'd like you to have them. When you see something you want that belongs to someone else, draw a picture of it. At the end of the day you can show me your pictures. We'll work out how you can get these things so you won't need to take them without the owner's permission." Ditty had not been given many presents, so receiving this gift gave her a warm feeling.

The next morning just before break, the teacher called Ditty over and put some lotion on her hands, suggesting, "Show your classmates how nice your hands smell and how soft they are!" Curiously, the other children gathered round, taking turns to smell Ditty's hands. Ditty loved having them being nice to her so she shared out the lotion. For two weeks, the teacher let the class put cream on each other's hands at break time. Ditty stopped scratching her classmates and made friends. She forgot how badly she needed other people's stuff and gave back most of the things she'd taken. Ditty drew a few pictures of things she liked but she no longer wanted them quite so badly. Now and again, out of habit, Ditty would scratch someone, but as her nails were softer they didn't hurt the person nearly as much. At home, Ma Domino told Ditty, "you're doing really well. I'm so proud of you!" Ditty felt much better.

Activities

- Make up a scrapbook: "All about me". Cut out or draw pictures of things you'd like and arrange them in the scrapbook.

- In pairs, rub lotion into each other's hands, place hands on paper, and dust with talcum powder; shake off surplus powder to reveal prints.

Materials

Scrapbooks, magazines and catalogues, glue, scissors, pens, sugar paper, non-allergenic hand lotion and talcum powder.

Discussion

- How do you think Ditty was feeling when she scratched her classmates? Might she be bored, angry or jealous of them?

- Why would Ditty want things that belonged to the other children?
  How do you feel if someone takes your things? Has that happened?

- Why do you think the teacher was worried about Ditty?

- How did the hand cream help Ditty to make friends?

- Was it a good idea to ask Ditty to draw the things she wanted?

- How would you like the story to continue or conclude?

Reflections

- Ditty was feeling jealous of her peers, who seemed to have all the things she wanted. She was also bored from not understanding what she should be doing in the lesson.

- As a neglected child, Ditty had very few valuable items of her own but wants to be the same as her classmates and own the same things.

- Her classmates are likely to resent Ditty taking their things. Some of them would be scared of her.

- The teacher was worried that Ditty wasn't getting on with her classmates. This was making it harder for her to concentrate and learn.

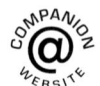

- The sensory and physical experience of spreading hand cream on the classmates' hands gave Ditty an opportunity to win back their trust and friendship.

- Giving Ditty the drawing book to draw pictures of things she wanted gave her permission to express her desire for particular things and work towards obtaining them legitimately.

- Ditty could be encouraged to take up a special interest to help sustain friendships.

Fear of school

Children, who have been taken away from their birth family because of neglect and abuse, are often highly anxious about the move to a new school (Luke et al., 2014). The loss of friendships formed in their previous school is likely to heighten their anxiety. Moves to a new adoptive or foster placement sometimes occur mid term, which can make the transition to another school especially difficult for the child. The child's caregivers and teachers could arrange a farewell visit for the child to see friends at their last school and ensure the child is able to access support staff when they need it.

For fostered and adopted children, the move to secondary school (usually between the ages of 11 and 13 years) also brings new challenges. The larger size of most secondary schools can feel intimidating. The teachers will be expecting their students to act more responsibly, demonstrate a social conscience (for example, by picking up their litter and being polite) and to respond to social signals such as making eye contact when spoken to. The inability to read social cues may present as lack of cooperation and raise anxiety in teachers who do not yet know the child or their background.

Story 11, "Della's difficulties", describes the fears of a fostered girl, who is moving to a new secondary school. Della is encouraged to practise dealing with unwelcome taunts in fictional contexts. This gives her the confidence to adjust and cope better in real-life situations. It also alleviated her fears of being bullied, put down, or being unable to manage her academic work.

How to use this story

- Parents, social workers, teaching staff and counsellors can read Story 11 as a means to discuss school-based worries with the child. It is important to give anxious children a sense of hope that they can cope.

- The child can be invited to rehearse assertive responses with the adult, in order to alleviate their fears of being bullied and told off or put down.

- Help the child to make a list of assertive responses, which they can keep with them to re-read in private, should they need to use them.

- Dramatise fictional situations in which bullying occurs, to enable the children to rehearse their responses. This will increase their confidence for coping with the predicaments they most dread.

- For children arriving mid term, ensure access to support staff, who can arrange visits to their last school to ease transition wherever possible.

Story 11: Della's difficulties

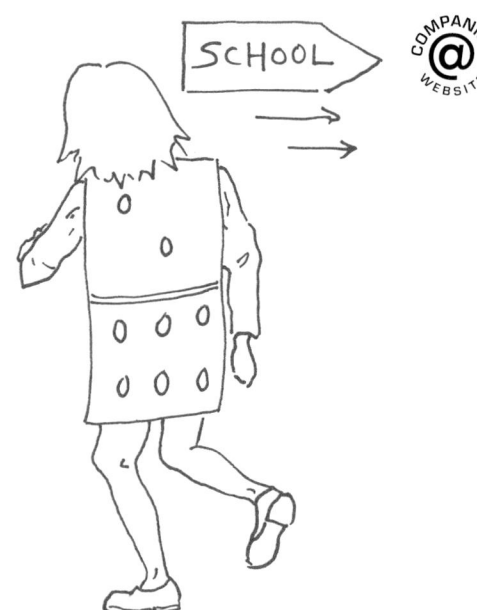

Della had been living at Ma Domino's for a few years. Now aged 12, she was about to move to secondary school and really dreaded it. As the school was so much bigger than she was used to, Della was scared of getting lost finding her way to classes. She worried about losing things and being given a hard time, even though she couldn't help it. Della expected the work to be too hard and that she'd be given loads of homework. Her worst worry was that she'd meet people from the first school she went to, who would remember her from her birth family. Suppose they said something she couldn't handle? Her foster brothers and sisters went to this secondary school. Della knew they'd tease her or say dumb things likely to make other people see her as weird. Ma Domino reassured her, "don't worry they'll look after you!" But just thinking about it made Della's tummy twist itself into knots. Ma Domino knew Della was scared so she suggested, "Let's think of ways you can protect yourself." The first idea they came up with was to ignore silly remarks – shrug, turn your back and walk away. Next, they made a list of places where Della could escape to, such as the library or music practice room.

They thought of responses to nasty taunts:

"Get lost!"

"It takes one to know one!"

"I'm so glad I don't think the way you do!"

"It's a shame that all you can talk about is a load of rubbish!"

"If that's how you think, your mind must be a sewer!"

"Well, time's moved on and so have I. Shame I can't say the same about you!"

"You think you're so funny, you should just listen to yourself!"

"I'm so glad this doesn't worry me like it seems to bother you!"

Ma Domino wrote these responses on a set of cards for Della to keep in her bag. Della realised that if she got into a situation that made her feel scared, she could look for a friend or a teacher she trusted and ask for help. Or she could stay silent, or buy herself time by saying she had to meet someone. To avoid getting drawn into doing stupid dares, Della practised sounding confident, saying things like, "No way! I don't want to be grounded!"

They rehearsed several situations and strategies then discussed the reactions they each got. Della noticed that when the "victim" turned her back, the bully's responses had less effect. But then she reasoned, "If I walk off, they might think they'd won and come after me." Ma Domino admitted this was a risk and advised her, "If you get bullied, I want to know about it. I'll report it because your teachers have a responsibility to stop the misuse of power."

Ma Domino suggested that Della draw round her hand on a piece of card, then write on each card finger, the names of people and places she could go to, if she found herself in a situation that made her feel anxious. Ma Domino reminded her, "Even if you don't have your cards with you, you always have your hand so when you look at it you'll remember where you can go for help."

Della visited the new school and was given a timetable and map of the classrooms with subject labels on each room. She didn't get lost because on her first day there, she made a friend who was doing nearly all the same subjects as her so they went to classes, together. The massive size of the school meant that the older dominoes had different break times so Della hardly ever saw her brothers and sisters, which was one less worry.

Della saw two students from her old school and was ready in case it turned into a problem but she noticed that one of them was looking wide and heavy. The other one's dots were discoloured. Della reckoned they'd be too scared of retaliation to risk making nasty comments about her. After three weeks, neither of them said anything about the past, so Della stopped worrying.

The work turned out to be not as hard as she'd feared. The teachers were pleased with her efforts and gave her credits, so she relaxed and made some more friends. Della loved animals and wanted to work with a vet. Now she was hopeful of good enough marks to get this kind of work when she's older.

Activities

- In pairs, share ideas and write advice sheets for coping with school.

- Each young person can draw round her hand on a piece of card, then write on each card finger, the names of people and places she could go to, if she found herself in a situation that made her feel anxious.

- Using Worksheet 2, make up your own responses to taunts.

- In small groups, act out the following scenes and decide what should happen in each of these situations, then discuss arising feelings.

- *In the playground, a group of girls are teasing someone.*

- *A teacher makes an unflattering comparison between a brother and sister.*

- *A student accuses a boy of cheating.*

Materials

Cards, pens and crayons.

Discussion

- Why might Della be scared of going to her new school? Do you find the students or teachers scary? What do you dread (or like) at school?

- What kind of taunts do you think Della was expecting? How might you help a mate who was in Della's situation?

- Changing school can make anyone anxious. Can you think what would help you prepare for this situation?

- Sometimes children dread being compared with their siblings. How might brothers or sisters help or hinder you at school?

Reflections

- Della's dread of being unable to cope in her new school is typical of lots of children in foster, adoptive and kinship families.

- She was afraid that she might be bullied by other students and that teachers would tell her off for being unable to keep up with the work.

- It is important to invite children in such a situation to talk about their worries.

- Della was scared of being called a "loser" "minger" or worse. Making a friend helped her feel braver and more confident.

- Giving new students a map of the classrooms helps them find their way around school. Teachers can ask students to befriend the newcomer.

- Parents can help the child prepare for going to a new school by practising what to say in the situations their child most dreads.

- Parents can also help a child maintain contact with important friendships from their last school.

Hiding

It is common for children to blame themselves for abuse and rejection in their highly traumatic past (de Thierry, 2017). Many continue to do so for every unfortunate thing that happens to them. Some children will have had to take responsibility for looking after younger siblings. Neglect often means little or no training in self-care and extreme anxiety makes it even harder to keep control of bodily functions, evidence of which the child may conceal. Their hiding of food or soiled clothing indicates the child is too scared to risk facing the disgust and embarrassment of asking what to do about it. Wearing unwashed clothes makes it difficult for children to find friends and feel welcomed in social activities. This reinforces their sense of inadequacy and self-hatred. Story 12, "Dilys blames herself" shows how a parent's constant criticism led the child to believe it all and despise herself. It illustrates how Dilys was helped to gain a sense of pride as a survivor of debilitating trauma.

How to use the story:

- Invite the child to try out the suggested creative activities. She might not want to talk about her worries, which may feel too embarrassing for her.

- Reassure her that children are not to blame for circumstances, which lead them to being taken into care. It is up to adults to keep children safe.

- Explain that Dilys had been given unrealistic levels of responsibility.

- Ask why Dilys blamed herself, lived in fear, and what kind of social activities might encourage her to join in and make friends.

- Help children feel more confident about asking for help when they need it.

Story 12: Dilys blames herself

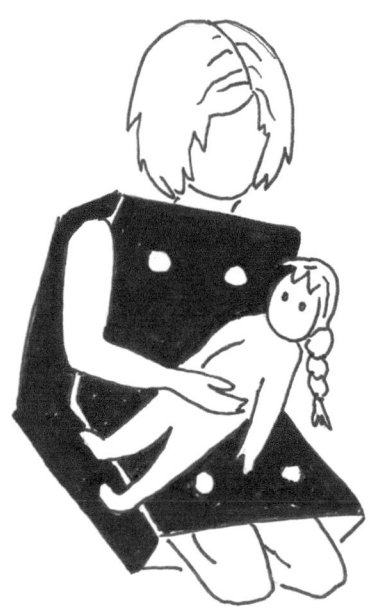

Dilys, aged 10, hated herself. When anything went wrong, she took the blame, always assuming it was her fault even when it blatantly wasn't. Dilys was scared of being told off in case she got chucked out of Ma Domino's. Even though she'd lived there for ages, she wasn't sure how to use the shower so avoided it and hid her dirty clothes. Dilys had been to lots of foster families, who had asked for her to be moved on. Before that, when she was living with her birth Mum, their bath was always full of dirty laundry, which meant they never got the chance to wash themselves in it. Her birth Mum was mentally ill and constantly harped on at Dilys for doing things wrong like not changing her baby sister's nappy correctly, even though Dilys was still a child. Ma Domino worried when she noticed that Dilys avoided activities she'd tried to get her involved in to help her make friends. The snag was, Dilys felt picked on by the other girls so, sensing she wasn't wanted, she dropped out of each of these activities as soon as she could.

One day in the school holidays the other dominoes went on an outing. Dilys didn't want to go so she stayed behind. An idea came to Ma Domino, who brought out some dolls, a toy bath, dolls' nappies and lotion. She asked Dilys to help her sort out a pile of dolls clothes. As soon as Dilys saw the nappies she went stiff and said, "I can't!" but couldn't explain why. Calmly Ma Domino said, "Ok, just watch and you can help if I get stuck". They worked out which outfits fitted which doll then Ma Domino began to wash and dress the dolls. Some of the clothes were a tight fit. As Ma struggled to dress a life-size doll, Dilys instinctively moved its arm to make the sleeve fit. Ma Domino said, "Thanks Dilys, that's really helpful! Can you do the next one for me?" Dilys took the doll from her, bathed it and added some lotion then put a nappy on it as she'd seen Ma Domino do. "Well done! You're a natural!" said Ma Domino. Unable to believe her, Dilys replied, "No I'm not! I'm rubbish at everything!" Ma Domino said, "You only think that because you believed your birth Mum. But she was so unwell she wouldn't know how unkind she was being. If that doll was a real baby, he'd be very pleased to have you looking after him."

Ma Domino took Dilys to the supermarket and let her pick her favourite shower gel and shampoo. Back at home Dilys was persuaded to try them out and Ma Domino showed her how the shower worked. Dilys began to feel less scared of water and to enjoy having showers. Ma Domino arranged for Dilys to leave school early once a week so she could play with the baby dolls while the others were out. Gradually, encouraged by Ma Domino, Dilys began to create stories of mums being kind to their babies. Some days they took the dolls to the park and put them on the swings. At school the other children stopped avoiding her and one girl came and sat next to her. When a new girl came to the school, the teacher asked Dilys to look after her. Scared the new girl wouldn't like her Dilys told Ma Domino about it. Ma Domino said, "I'm sure she will like you. You are kind and a good friend. I'm so proud of you!" The next day, Dilys spent the break talking to the new girl, who was glad to have someone be kind to her. They made friends and Dilys felt much happier.

Activities

- Wash and dress dolls and apply lotion. Massage lotion on your own hands. How does this feel? What do you think of the smell?

- Create a story, in which a problem gets resolved.

- Try out different scents and spray a favourite scent onto a small piece of material to keep and smell when you feel anxious.

- Draw and colour in pictures of activities that you missed out on like feeding ducks in the park, going to the seaside, or the zoo.

- With the family make a play and act out these activities.

Materials

Dolls, bath, baby lotion, scented shower gel, paper and crayons.

Discussion

- Do you think children often blame themselves when things go wrong?

- How does it feel to suffer repeated criticism?

- Is it fair to give children responsibility for younger siblings?

- Have you ever had to look after your siblings? What was it like?

- What helped Dilys to enjoy showers?

- How did Ma Domino help Dilys?

- How did the teacher help?

Reflections

- It is natural to blame yourself when you feel unwanted and things go wrong. Constant criticism from her birth Mum left Dilys believing any bad things said to her. She had lots of fears and very low self-esteem.

- Children should never be given responsibility for the tasks of feeding, bathing and changing younger siblings. Yet when parents are mentally unwell their children take on these responsibilities all too frequently.

- Ma Domino encouraged Dilys to face her fears through play with baby dolls. Choosing her favourite scents encouraged Dilys to enjoy using them in the shower.

- The teacher was empathic, allowing Dilys time out of school for therapeutic play.

3 The legacy of mental illness

Most children in adoptive, kinship or foster families will have experienced neglect, abuse and family breakdown, all of which are immensely traumatic and frequently lead to complex problems in adjustment. The legacy of mental illness can last a lifetime. It affects the children's future relationships, their emotional well-being and capacity to learn and make best use of education. The poor outcomes for affected children evidence the need for improved services with more creative approaches to address these children's needs.

This chapter reflects on the particular experience in foster, kinship and adoptive families, of children whose birth parents are mentally ill. Half of the children and young people in local authority care now meet the criteria for mental health diagnosis (DfE, 2018). Children, who have been exposed to domestic violence, are particularly likely to continue to suffer symptoms of post-traumatic stress disorder. Many, who are troubled by low self-esteem, self-harm and suffer from body dysmorphia and eating disorder.

These stories illustrate how appropriate adult interaction helps young people to experience compassion, comfort, solace, and feel understood in order that they can better adjust and find ways to deal with their predicament. The suggestions for creative activities are to guide the involved adult to help the young people find their own solutions.

Parents' mental illness

Parents' depression, psychosis and personality disorder influence the genetic makeup, attachment security and behavioural development of their children (Manning and Gregoire, 2009), increasing their vulnerability (Kelly and McBride, 2019). Mentally ill parents often blame children unfairly for their problems. Children almost invariably accept the blame, believing the unkind things said to them. As they grow up and approach adolescence, they lack the model they need to manage relationships successfully. Looking after parents and younger siblings places them at risk of missing out on educational and social activities and falling victim to embarrassing, stigmatising jibes. At the pre-teen stage, many become anxious about inheriting their parents' illness and need to know that receiving good care substantially reduces this risk.

We can enable children in the foster, kinship and adoptive care of securely attached adults to recover nurture and the opportunities they missed out on. It is important for the involved adults to avoid unhelpful blame and shame of birth parents whose choices were limited. After all, the children are likely to be highly sensitive to any inference or hint of criticism of their birth parent and may feel that they too, must therefore be "faulty". Story 13 "Dodgems" illustrates the anxieties and sense of guilt preying on two children, who run away from their mentally ill mother. The story conveys permission for them to love the substitute parents as well as their birth parents. Sensitively exploring the fears that the children have experienced helps them to feel less isolated.

How to use the story

- Read story 13. Explain that Del and Dorca feel guilty about having abandoned their mentally ill birth mother at home. They also worry about what might happen if she finds out where they are living.

- Keeping to the context of the story, talk about what helps children to cope, such as having friends or knowing what to do in tricky situations.

- Use costumes, puppets or toys to dramatise scenes from Story 13 or allow the child or children to develop their own story.

- In reference to the story's description of frightening experience, clarify that children are not to blame for a parent's problems but are entitled to be cared for, educated, given good food and clothing, time to rest, spend time with friends and study, in order to achieve their future ambitions.

- Improvise stories such as *Cinderella* and *Aladdin*. The children's dramatisations may serve to illustrate how very differently life turns out when a person feels cared about and emotionally supported.

- Scenes from "Dodgems" can lead into exploring children's fears that they might turn out to be like their birth parents and cope poorly in life.

- Explain that with good care Del and Dorca will be making better choices. For example Ma Domino reassures them (that their birth mother was now far away) encourages them to feel safer with her.

- Adoptive parents, foster parents and teachers can take this opportunity to convey that tactless, unkind remarks are unacceptable. Encourage the children to practise ignoring or challenging this unpleasantness.

Story 13: Dodgems

Del and his sister, Dorca, had run away from home because their mentally ill birth Mum was so scared of being on her own they'd had to stay off school to look after her. She stopped taking her medicine and kept cutting her arms. The police came and took Del and Dorca to Ma Domino's. All that happened a few months ago. Today it was Dorca's 13th birthday. The young Dominoes had come to the fairground as a birthday treat. First, they all headed to the ghost train. Most of the dominoes loved it but Del and Dorca were unnerved by the ghostly figures looming up and reminding them of scary people they knew. When it stopped Del headed over to the dodgems. As they weaved around, he bumped into a boy, who accused him of doing it deliberately, but Del wasn't but it made him very anxious.

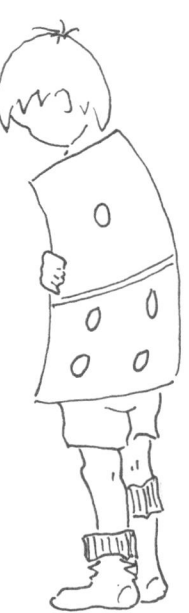

Next, they piled on to the merry-go-round. The pods spanning round made a kaleidoscope of colour. Dorca loved the way the images blended until the ride slowed down. Then heaps of litter reminded her of mess they'd left behind. Guilt made her feel queasy – scared she'd turn out like Mum. Del yelled: "What'll we go on now?" He'd spotted the swing boat, which had a brilliant view from the high end. But Dorca was heading to the roller coaster. Del didn't want to be on his own so he rushed to catch her up. The coaster moved fast, clanking like mad. Del wasn't at all sure he was brave enough to go on it. Dorca looked a bit green but scoffed, "Bet you ain't got the nerve!" Del replied "I have an' all!" She sniggered, "Na, you're chicken!" Del thumped her. He was scared but daren't admit it. As the coaster slowed to a halt, the queue began moving so Del had to make up his mind. Sensing that if he showed any weakness he'd get dissed, reluctantly, he climbed in. As they got strapped in, Dorca asked him, "You OK?" Del shrugged, saying "This is boring, pathetic I reckon!" Dorca jeered, "Get off it then!" Del knew it was his last chance. His stomach knotted and he longed to bolt, but his pride wouldn't let him.

The music started and the coaster gathered pace quickly. The climb upwards was ok, but coming down at lightening speed made Del feel sick. As the coaster rattled upwards and thundered down an old song was being played. It reminded Del of home and the fights when Dad drunkenly hit Mum and made her face stream with blood. Del had hidden. Now tears pricked the back of his eyes. He flushed with shame at his cowardice in not fighting Dad off. Since then Mum had met more creepy friends, whom he tried to avoid. Suddenly, the carriage plummeted down so fast he threw up.

Massive lumps of sick floated off on the wind, landing like a shower on people below. Lots of kids started screaming. Del's head thudded. The whole ride took four minutes but it felt like an eternity. The worst part was Dorca being kind to him – it was so humiliating that he swore at her. She marched off, crying. Del felt guilty – if only she'd just sneered, it wouldn't have mattered how nastily he'd reacted.

Hearing about the commotion, Ma Domino hurried towards them, exclaiming, "Well you've had some excitement, haven't you!" She'd brought spare clothes in case they got soaked on a water ride. Tactfully she steered Del towards the toilets to get changed. When he came back, she led them to a café, asking, "Did you have a lovely time?" Everyone described thrilling rides except for Del and Dorca, who fell silent. Suddenly Dorca announced, "I think I saw Mum!" Del glared at her and kicked her leg under the table. Dorca protested "I was only saying it looked like her!" They loved their Mum but were terrified that if she found them, their life would turn upside down again. It had been bad enough when Dad was around but at least, he'd made Mum take her pills. After he'd walked out on them, she kept talking to people, who weren't there and insisting bad things were happening even when they weren't. Sometimes when they were out in public Mum cried yet didn't say what was bothering her. It was embarrassing! She'd try and manipulate them or lose it completely.

Del and Dorca heard Ma Domino telling them, "There's no need to worry! Your Mum has been so poorly she's back in hospital. She's coming out soon but has moved away. We'll arrange for you to see her when you feel ready!" Relieved, Del and Dorca began to join in the conversation with the others.

Activities

- Make a fairground game: On a large piece of card draw and colour in pictures of rides and stalls selling toffee apples, candy floss or burgers. Divide the card into squares, numbered 1–50. Draw snakes and ladders.

- Play the fairground game, using dice, throwing a six to start at the square number one, and aim to get to the square numbered 50.

- Dramatise a scene from the story. Talk about the highs and lows of real life situations that the rides remind you of. Decide which failures in life represent the "snakes" and which highpoints are the "ladders".

Materials

Card, crayons, pens, rulers, dice.

Discussion

- The children's Mum must have felt terribly unhappy, to harm herself. What would you guess Del and Dorca worried about most?

- Sounds, sights and smells can bring back memories of the past. Who might ghostly figures remind the children of?

- How did their birth Mum embarrass Del?

- Why didn't Del want to show any weakness? What made him so angry with himself for being scared to go on the roller coaster ride? What fairground ride do you find scariest? Does it make you sick?

- Dorca thought she saw her birth Mum. It can be worrying to sense you've seen someone from the past. How did Ma Domino help?

- The likelihood of inheriting a parent's mental illness is statistically, tiny, especially if you are being looked after properly. What do you think? What kind of support do children need from parents?

- Why might children love parents who are too ill to meet their needs? Do you think its ok to love people who are not your birth parents?

Reflections

- Del and Dorca felt under too much strain to cope with their mother's mental illness as it kept them from school. They felt upset and afraid that she'd overdose and make them responsible for the outcome.

- The ghostly figures may have been reminders of their Dad, or of their Mum's subsequent partners, who frightened and abused her and them.

- The children's mother had hallucinations and would talk to people she imagined were present but were not actually there. She cried in public without giving any explanation.

- Sometimes children worry that if they display any weakness, others will exploit it and attack them for it. Del was anxious to avoid it. He daren't show his fear of the roller coaster in case he got mocked for it.

- Ma Domino explained that their Mum had been looked after in hospital and since then, had moved to another part of the country. Ma Domino reassured them that she would take them to visit their Mum, but only when they felt ready for this.

- Children rely on parents to meet all their needs – for food, clothing, shelter, opportunities to play, study and learn, to develop interests and ambitions and have rewarding relationships.

- Love has no limits. This means it is possible to love two sets of parents without being disloyal to either.

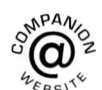

Domestic violence

A UK government commissioned report (Stanley, 2011) found domestic violence occurring most often alongside social and economic disadvantage, which causes stress and frequently interacts with factors of poor mental health, substance misuse and homelessness. A substantial proportion of children in foster, kinship and adoptive families will have witnessed domestic violence. The silence that follows such incidents is especially frightening. Violence between parents arouses fear, anxiety, worry and anger in their children. The sense of isolation and stigma is compounded when a parent is mentally ill. The risk of psychological harm to their children increases if they also experience other forms of abuse and neglect. Daily occurrence of abuse and neglect affects how children view themselves and those around them. Van der Kolk (2015), Shonkoff and Levitt (2010) and Teicher (2016) find that the neurological patterns in brains of traumatised children differ from the norm.

Practitioners need to be skilled in talking directly to children about their experience of domestic violence, listen to them and validate their accounts. Children's relationships and possessions form a strong part of their identity. Children who are taken in to foster care and go on to have further moves, suffer losses that include their sense of identity and self, which for traumatised children are already fragmented. The fifth stage of grieving that Kubler Ross (1969) identifies as "acceptance", is in my experience, difficult to reach for abused children, who find it exceptionally difficult to trust anyone. Story 14 illustrates the predicament for a child struggling with loss and change.

"Dilly feels silly" is about an 11-year-old girl left bereft by her mother's death, following her father's incarceration. Being listened to and supported alleviates her sense of isolation. It is important to validate children's memories and reflect on their courage in surviving adversity and still coping day to day.

How to use the story

- Read the story and improvise scenes from it.

- Use creative activities to invite children to talk about their feelings.

- Some children may be keen to enact scenes from their own life story. School counsellors and adoptive/foster parents are advised to check the accuracy of the children's memories with the social worker's knowledge of the history and ask for answers to children's questions.

- To avoid breach of confidentiality in school, it is best to use fictional stories. It is imperative to avoid the re-enactment of violence or other frightening events. Playing the scene of the "morning after" such events (rather than the event itself) will avert the risk of re-traumatisation.

- In dramatic play the social worker or therapist might invite the child to take the role of the "birth parent". In this role the child may change the outcome and make different decisions to those of their birth parents.

- Help the children appreciate that having better care enables them to make progress and avoid self-blame for past rejection.

- Encourage children to reconstruct their self-image positively and feel pride. Acknowledge their courage and ability to love others.

- Discuss the experience for children, who witnessed fights and missed out on proper care and education, to which all children are entitled.

Story 14: Dilly feels silly

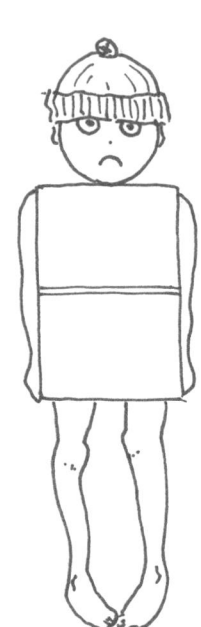

Dilly, aged 11, came from a travelling family, who moved around the country. This meant Dilly hadn't been to any school for long. When she did go, she hardly ever made friends. Some children called her "pikey" and said no one liked being seen with her. Dilly's parents frequently fought, which had made her life stressful. Her Mum wasn't allowed off site on her own. Often when Dad wasn't around, Mum got another man to take her to the shops and flirted with him, as a wind up. When Dad heard about it he got so jealous, he gave her "what for" as he called it. Things got much worse after he'd been drinking. Dilly was usually in bed by the time the rows started but she still heard everything. The silence that followed them was the scariest of all. One night, Mum got injured so badly, she had to be taken to hospital. The police locked Dad up. When Mum left the hospital, they went to unlicensed sites and Mum spent most evenings in the pub. She stopped getting up in the morning, which meant Dilly missed even more school. Eventually, the authorities caught up with them and took Dilly to Ma Domino's.

Mum put off visiting Dilly in her new home and carried on drinking. Before long, her liver packed up and she died. What most upset Dilly was finding out that her Mum had been staying nearby yet had not come to see her. Dilly ached to see her Mum. It was bad enough waiting so long but now she would never see her. Everyone expected Dilly to carry on as normal, but she kept half expecting her Mum to appear. This made it impossible to concentrate. Dilly was always losing things or forgetting where she was. She didn't have any of her Mum's stuff, not even a photo. It was horribly upsetting when her mental image of Mum began blurring and slipping away. Dilly felt as though she'd lost everything and no longer had any sense of who she was.

At school, the others didn't know that Dilly's Mum had just died. They only noticed her mistakes, which were hardly surprising since Dilly had been out of school more days than in it. Their jokes didn't help. When Dilly didn't answer questions or follow teachers' instructions, the teachers got annoyed and told her off while her classmates giggled, calling her "Silly Dilly!" One day was especially bad. Getting picked on was embarrassing and made Dilly feel hopeless, like she'd never do anything right. Back at Ma Dominos, she cried as if she'd never stop. Ma patted her gently and tried to reassure her. After a while, she asked Dilly if she could remember any nice times with her family, before her Dad went to prison. Dilly talked about looking after horses so Ma Domino took her to a field where horses were grazing.

"Go on", she said. As Dilly stroked the horses, she remembered other nice times, like playing dominos, doing hopscotch and Auntie Mo teaching her how to ride a bike.

Dilly loved drawing so Ma Domino gave her a book to draw her memories in. Dilly cried again but now she felt comforted. Each day, she drew pictures of her old life. She told Ma about Auntie Mo, who had tried to protect her. When Ma Domino discovered that Dilly's Auntie Mo had moved nearby she began taking Dilly for visits. Auntie Mo was so impressed by Dilly's pictures, she suggested taking them into school. When the teacher saw the pictures she put some on the wall. Another day she invited the class to draw their earliest memories. One girl got upset. Dilly told her that she too, missed her Mum. After that, her class stopped calling her "Silly Dilly" and Dilly made friends.

Activities

- Write and decorate a poem about a person (or a pet) you loved.

- Make a collage of photos and drawings of a person or pet you miss.

- Using Worksheet 3 draw and colour your memories in a memory jar.

- Draw a picture of a rocket going into space. Write a list of things you would like to do with someone you feel close to.

- Light a candle, pretend it's the person you miss and say the things you'd want them to know about how you feel if they were still around.

Materials

Worksheet 3, paper, pens, crayons, collage materials, photos.

Discussion

- The story describes difficulties affecting travelling children. How does it feel to keep moving home and not see your friends from the last place?

- It is often hard for children when parents split up. Dilly's father went to prison. How do you think parental violence affects their children?

- Dilly's Mum died from heavy drinking. When parents use illegal drugs or drink too much alcohol, what does it feel like for their children?

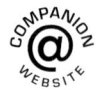

- How did Dilly experience being taken to a family that wasn't part of her travelling community? Was she upset or relieved or both? I wonder why Dilly's Mum didn't visit her at Ma Domino's.

- Dilly was very upset by her Mum's death and kept expecting her to appear. Has this happened to you? How did it affect you?

- Dilly felt silly when she kept forgetting or losing her things. Has that happened to you? How does it make you feel if people scoff at you?

- Why do you think Dilly felt she was losing her sense of identity?

- How did Ma Domino and Auntie Mo help Dilly? What advice would you give Dilly?

- Shall we write the next chapter? Might Dilly move in with Auntie Mo?

Reflections

- Some travelling families move regularly from site to site across counties. This disrupts children's schooling and makes it hard for them to maintain friendships. It can leave them feeling left out and excluded.

- Travelling children are all too often stigmatised for the anti-social behaviour of adults in their community, and having a parent in prison.

- Parental violence is frightening for a child to witness. Dilly was likely to have sleep problems and anxiety from expecting the violence to repeat. She would be anticipating that the victim will get even more damaged.

- Heavy use of drugs and alcohol can make parents too poorly to look after their children, who then have to look after themselves. Being left to their own devices puts them in danger of accidents, scalds etc.

- Dilly had to get used to a different lifestyle, new expectations and rules. Trying to remember all the things expected of her raised her anxiety. She felt scared she would never fit in at school and worried about her Mum.

- Dilly's Mum may have been embarrassed to face people looking after Dilly, ashamed of her inability to stop drinking. Or she may have been too taken up with her own needs to even think about Dilly's feelings.

- Loss of a parent is very distressing. Dilly felt deserted. Such a loss disrupts the brain's memory systems and makes it harder for the child to concentrate and deal with all the demands of day-to-day life. The problem gets worse when we get derided for our mistakes.

- Having no picture of her Mum left Dilly struggling to remember what she looked like. Already separated from her travelling community, she was scared she'd lost her sense of identity and where she belonged.

- Ma Domino helped Dilly by listening with compassion and comforting her through her distress. Finding out where Dilly's aunt lived enabled Dilly to rebuild her relationship with her. Encouraging her to talk about her memories and develop her skills in drawing helped Dilly make friends.

- Dilly's Auntie Mo helped by praising Dilly for her artistic skills and suggesting she take her pictures into school.

- The children might develop the story by having Dilly move in with Auntie Mo and keep up the links with their community. Decide how supportive the community might be.

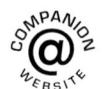

Post-traumatic stress disorder

Post-traumatic stress disorder (PTSD) affects many children in foster, kinship and adoptive families. It also affects unaccompanied refugee children, who, since 2015, have been arriving in the UK in unprecedented numbers from war torn countries (O'Higgins et al., 2018). The authorities tasked to care for them have struggled to know how best to meet their needs. For children parted from their family, friends and everything they know, unfamiliarity with the language adds to their sense of isolation, which is intensified by absence of shelter, food or comfort. In addition to material and practical needs, they need to be able to communicate and understand things such as the non-verbal signals used in their new environment. Peterson et al. (2017) advise that care and education is central to meeting their needs for inclusion and development. Story 15 illustrates the sense of powerlessness for a child, who is traumatised by wartime atrocities yet is enabled to create a new more secure life for herself. The story is to help children make sense of past experience and gain confidence to adjust to their new circumstances.

How to use the story

- Read the story and dramatise scenes from it.

- Talk about cultural differences in non-verbal communication between the home country of refugee children and where they live now.

- For children learning English as a new language and needing practice in using new words and phrases, have subtitles on the TV screen to enable them to read the words they hear spoken.

Story 15: Dixie's devastation

Dixie saw her father shot and mutilated. She'd escaped war in her homeland, not knowing if any of her family was still alive. Dixie felt guilty that she was alive when the rest of them could be dead. It was a long journey to Planet Domino and things happened that were so hideous, she tried to forget them. She knew no one here, where people spoke a different language. Dixie was starving, having not eaten for days. Seeing someone throw half a burger away, she picked it up and took a bite but it made her throw up. Hours later, Ma Domino found her slumped in a doorway. She lifted and half carried the sick girl back to her house.

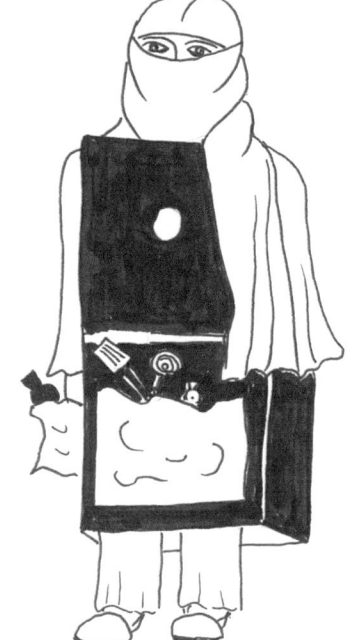

Ma Domino managed to get the authorities' permission to let Dixie stay. Dixie was glad of a bed, food and warm clothes. She was 14, so she had to go to school but as she didn't know the language, most of the time she couldn't join in conversations. The school had interpreters but they didn't come in every day. When teachers spoke to Dixie she avoided eye contact because where she came from it was rude to look adults in the eye. Discouraged, they gave up trying to help her. As soon as Dixie came out of school, people seemed to be shouting. Their hostility terrified her. At night she was scared to sleep since as soon as she did she had terrible nightmares and woke up screaming. During the day, sounds of a door slamming, a tin falling off a shelf, or someone shrieking, revived Dixie's memories of gunshots, people screaming and pools of blood, scenes that seemed to be happening to her in that moment. The sight of police uniforms left her rigid with fear but she couldn't tell anyone.

Ma Domino invited an interpreter to visit. This lady, who spoke Dixie's language listened to her then told Ma Domino what was happening in Dixie's home country, how her father got shot and why she came to Planet Domino. Ma Domino invited her niece, Dorrie, round. Dorrie drew a pictorial map for Dixie, to show the location of places like the advice centre where interpreters worked, the doctor's surgery, dentist, optician, library, cinemas and leisure club. Dixie had a good sense of direction and found the map very useful. She practised phrases in Domino language with the others in Ma's family. Within a few weeks, Dixie began to chat more easily and feel she was slotting in with the family. A few months later, an immigration official sent Ma Domino news of Dixie's brothers. The official still didn't know if their mother was alive, but Dixie was overjoyed to find out that her brothers were living nearby. Dixie looked forward to seeing them and began to feel more hopeful for the future.

Activities

- Walk round the room avoiding eye contact. Talk about how this feels. Talk in "gobbledy gook" and see if the others can guess what you are trying to say by observing your gestures and body language.

- On Worksheet 4, draw a map of your town or village, and pictures of places you go to such as shops, leisure centre and school.

- Act out the story of an unaccompanied child refugee. Make a list of things that would help the refugee adjust to their new life.

Materials

Stiff card and felt tip pens, access to on-line resources.

Discussion

- Do you know any child from a war torn country, or who suffers from terrifying flashbacks? What problems did they face?

- Can you guess what happened to Dixie on her way to Planet Domino?

- How does war affect children? Sometimes home life feels like war.

- What do children need? What help would you like to have?

- How hard is it to be unable to confide in anyone?

- How would you go about learning a new language?

- Why is it important to help vulnerable people?

Reflections

- Flashbacks are memories that lead the child to believe the event is occurring in that moment. The fear of its recurrence is paralysing.

- We often adapt to a new situation by repressing terrifying memories, pretending bad things didn't happen in order to help us stay in control.

- We can guess that Dixie met scary people who had terrified her. When she arrived she was starving but had no money for food and shelter.

- War can cause post-traumatic stress, which affects sleep, digestion, the ability to concentrate, memory retention and relationships. Experience of betrayal and fear of death makes it hard to trust anyone.

- Children can help someone like Dixie by being their friend. Child refugees, or children new to the school may need help to find their way around and understand expectations – deadlines for homework etc.

- It is bewildering for children when the people around them speak a different language and neither understands the other.

- Learning a new language takes time. It may help to make lists of the new words and phrases they learn each day and practise using them.

- Organisations such as the Salvation Army and Red Cross trace people; social workers may contact the police, Home Office and social media for information.

- It is important that children suffering from PTSD are supported in school, have access to therapeutic services, as well as to learning and opportunities to develop their skills, interests and friendships.

Self-harm

In preparing to move into adolescence, the need to try out new identities as individuals and as members of their peer group often becomes especially complicated for fostered and adopted children. Around 11–12 years of age, increased grey matter allows new connections to be made and brains to become ripe for risk taking. Inevitably the quest for independence involves making mistakes. Instances of self-harm have been steadily rising for the 10–14s (by at least 30% in the last decade). The process of maturation requires the child to begin to emotionally separate from parental influences but it is not helped by the availability of You Tube videos, which demonstrate risky behaviours such as choking, cutting and setting oneself on fire (Ahern et al., 2015). Whilst for most young people it is natural that feelings towards the opposite sex grow more powerful and exciting, acute self-consciousness makes the navigation of relationships fraught with anxiety. Heightened sensitivity, rejection, betrayal and experience of bullying flood them with intense emotions that threaten to overwhelm. Story 16 describes the crippling humiliation when unreciprocated passion replicates past rejection.

How to use this story

- Read and dramatise the story to provide practice at relationships, expressing emotions and using intuition intelligently.

- To reduce children's anxiety, explain that survival instincts help us to make rapid decisions to keep us safe when it is necessary.

- Ask how the problem arose and discuss strategies for dealing with it.

Story 16: Daffyd's desire

Daffyd, 13, was in love but the object of his desire didn't know it yet. This was Davina, who was in his class but new to the area, and still to get to know them all. Daffyd thought about Davina all the time. He dreamt of her blue eyes, her silky hair and scent. He imagined holding her and stroking her hair. The snag was that Daffyd couldn't think how to ask her out. He was terrified that if he did, she'd say no and might even laugh at him! For Daffyd, it felt much safer to hope she'd eventually like him than risk getting turned down because if that happened, he figured his life would no longer be worth living.

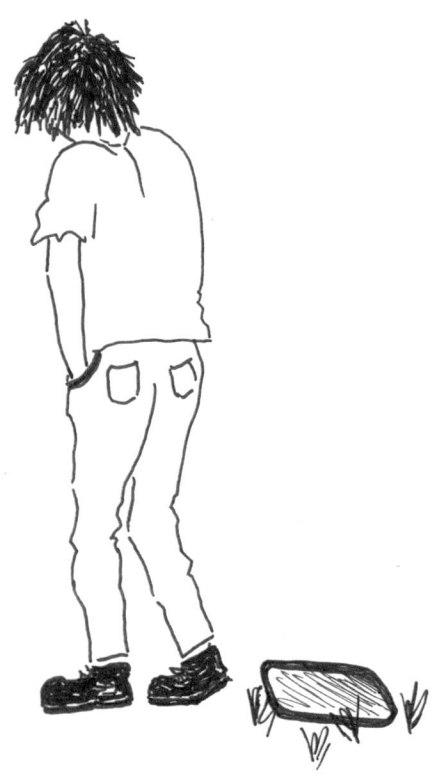

Daffyd became increasingly obsessed with Davina. Being good at art, he drew pictures of her. One day, during class, someone snatched his drawing and passed it to the girl next to him, whispering, "Guess what! Daffyd fancies Davina!" Daffyd felt his face flame up. Practically dying of embarrassment, he asked for it back, stuttering, "I'm just practising for art, that's all!" The other lad sniggered, "Funny, how you've gone all red then!" The drawing got passed on to Davina, who stared at it. The teacher asked her, "What's going on?" Breathlessly, Daffyd waited. Davina slipped the drawing into her folder, saying, "I was checking what we're meant to be doing." The teacher explained the task and moved on.

At break, Davina came looking for Daffyd and asked, "Why were you drawing me?" Daffyd couldn't think how to answer without sounding pathetic or idiotic. Davina said, "It's a really good picture only my boyfriend gets jealous and he won't like another guy coming on to me, ok?" Daffyd felt totally crushed and sick. A noise drummed in his ears, so loud, it drowned out the voices of the other girls asking him to draw pictures of them. Daffyd fled and hid behind the bins until the rest of the class went in. Then he walked out of school, believing he'd never get over the humiliation. Being very sensitive, Daffyd was an easy target so for the next few weeks, he went into school to get his attendance mark then slipped out and hung round the shops. Someone persuaded him to try a tablet that made him hallucinate. As the effects wore off, the

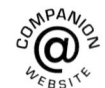

memory of his humiliation was so intense he began to punish himself by cutting the inside of his arms. At school, no one missed Daffyd until a teacher noticed that he hadn't handed in his homework and rang Ma Domino to ask why.

Daffyd had lived at Ma Domino's for several years. His Dad was violent to his Mum and when she escaped, he'd turned on Daffyd. His Mum never came back for him. Aching for her, he dreamed that if only she knew where he was she'd come for him. Daffyd tried to contact her on Facebook but got no reply. He felt no one cared if he existed. Ma Domino was kind but always busy with such a large family. Even so she had noticed Daffyd's misery and was worried about him. That evening, during dinner, she asked everyone in the family to say things they liked and admired about Daffyd, who was amazed to hear the nice things they said. He went red, but this time with relief as he enjoyed the warmth and kindness they showed him, by inviting him to their clubs and offering to share their games and stuff. Later, Ma Domino talked to Daffyd about his birth parents. Her explanations helped him to stop blaming himself for the past. Daffyd went back to school feeling anxious but Davina and her friends were kind to him. He found he could enjoy just being mates with them.

Activities

- In discussing Daffyd's experience and reactions decide what could happen in the next chapter of the story.

- Draw (or find) a picture to represent each of the characters and paste it onto card. Make a small stand by cutting slits (of same length) in the middle of the figure's base and the top edge of the stand. Slide the base end of the figure into the stand, so that it stands up by itself.

- Use these card figures to act out scenes from the story from the points of view of Davina, her boyfriend and/or another classmate.

- In dramatic play practise ways to ask someone to come out with you.

Materials

Teen magazines, card, glue, scissors; an example to show the child or group.

Discussion

- What did being in love feel like for Daffyd? Do you think he was justified in being scared he'd be turned down?

- How do you decide whether or when to ask someone to be your boyfriend or girlfriend? At what age does this usually start?

- How might it feel to have no partner if all your mates have one? What do you think of Davina's response to the picture Daffyd drew?

- Should the teacher have been more helpful? If so, how?

- What sensations do you notice when you feel scared?
  What helps you to survive the experience?

- Can you think of other humiliating situations affecting your age group?
  How do you handle them and protect yourself?

- Why do you think Daffyd cut his arms?

- In what other ways do young people self-harm?
  What does it achieve? How can they be helped?

- If you were offered a tablet and didn't know what it was, what would you do? Can you say "No" and walk away if you feel under pressure to go along with the group? Shall we practise ways to say "No"?

- How did Ma Domino help Daffyd? What else might help?
  Can boys be friends with girls without it becoming too intense?

- What would you like to happen in the next chapter of this story?

Reflections

- Daffyd was born into a family embroiled in domestic violence. His Mum then abandoned him. This left him with poor self-belief and fear of being mocked and judged to be an idiot.

- Being in love was exciting for Daffyd, but left him extremely anxious about the risk of rejection and scorn. The age you ask someone to be your boy/girlfriend depends on whether you want a friend or sexual relationship. Platonic relationships are less demanding.

- It can feel embarrassing or isolating to be the only one in your peer group who has no girl/boyfriend. Teachers need to be ready to protect the most vulnerable children. Dafydd's teacher could have arranged support from someone with responsibility for pastoral care.

- To help children with traumatic memories to notice bodily sensations when they feel anxious ask them if they feel hot, ready to run, or hear drumming in their ears etc. This will give them time to think and find a safe place until they can talk to someone who knows their predicament.

- Any kind of bullying can prompt fragile victims to self-harm. It is important to maintain policies for protecting children from bullying. Practising giving various excuses prepares children for extricating themselves from the threat of bullying threatening their sense of safety.

- The child who injures himself by cutting probably feels desperate. Self-harm is often a cry for help and may include eating disorder. It can serve to draw attention to the child's need for emotional support.

- Talking about his life story helped Daffyd to stop blaming himself and gain confidence from realising he was a courageous survivor.

Body dysmorphia and eating disorder

Young people, who develop body dysmorphia and/or eating disorder, are often very unhappy and subject of bullying, or other misguided influence. Matthews et al. (2019) find early trauma prevalent in looked after and adopted children experiencing body dysmorphia, perhaps due to identity confusion. The most common eating disorders are "anorexia nervosa" (affecting 1–2% of the overall population, which results from the obsession to lose weight and a refusal to eat); and "bulimia nervosa" (binge-eating followed by self-induced vomiting and fasting). Starving the body of food changes the brain cells and consequently distorts young people's perception of their reflection. The young person may dispose of food by hiding it, take laxatives, exercise excessively and access websites giving irresponsible advice on ways to lose weight and deceive parents. If the young person's weight drops to below the centile for their age, GP referral is advised. Beat is a website that offers advice and support for young people with eating disorder. Story 17 "Dodie feels invisible" illustrates recovery from bulimia via a young person engaging in a photography project.

How to use the story

- View the disorder as a coping mechanism for dealing with problems to encourage the children to explore more appropriate ways forward.

- Ask self-critical children why they came to think so critically and who has made critical comments to them, before giving your view.

- Comparing photos can give the affected child a fresh perspective.

- Encourage them to aim for manageable size portions of favourite food.

- Invite their interest in others' problems and causes, to reduce the child's sense of isolation and to distract them from their anxieties.

Story 17: Dodie feels invisible

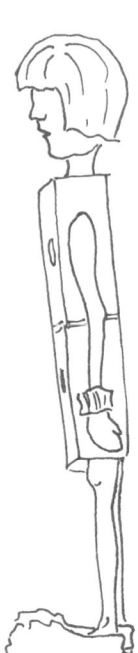

Dodie was thin and drained of colour. She was 13 and she was convinced that no one cared whether she lived or died. It all started when her Dad left the family several months back. Her Mum became depressed and ignored her so often that Dodie felt abandoned. At school, they'd been talking about all the things they wanted to do with their lives. Denise, who planned to be a model, said you had to get the right look or no one noticed you. She had fashionable clothes, stuff that most of them couldn't afford, which was annoying. Dodie was actually well proportioned but as they talked about their good and bad points, she confessed to being scared her thighs were too big. A boy they all fancied overheard her and yelled, "Meet Thunderthighs!" The other girls fell about laughing but Dodie felt totally humiliated.

That evening, as she stared into the mirror, Dodie saw herself as pure ugly. She wished she'd been born a boy and didn't have boobs sticking out in front. Her Mum rang to say she'd be late home again and told Dodie to get herself something from the freezer. Dodie warmed up a curry in the microwave and ate it, but then went to the toilet and threw up. After that she went online and found a website that gave tips on how to avoid eating and dispose of food discreetly. That summer, Dodie ate as little as possible. She passed bits of meat to the dog and stuck food behind the radiators. Yet the more weight she lost, the more dissatisfied she felt. To punish herself, Dodie scratched her wrists until they bled. She hoped the pain would mask other feelings, but it didn't. When the weather turned hot, she wore long sleeves so her Mum still didn't notice. Having no one she dared to confide in, Dodie cried and cried.

In September a new art teacher introduced the class to photography. Most of them loved it. But Dodie, believing she looked ugly, dreaded having her photo taken. She offered to help fetch supplies, a ploy that worked until the teacher noticed her lingering in the store cupboard and told her to join in. Dodie said, "I can't see the point, people will think I'm crap – I'll just take some photos of my friends." Guessing that Dodie was feeling horribly anxious, the teacher explained, "when you upload portrait photos, you can get rid of the parts you're not happy with and keep the image you like." She added, "You don't even have to smile – moody and melancholy can look just as good!" The teacher directed the group to take pictures of Dodie, who, given no choice, nervously posed for the camera. As her classmates admired the images they captured of her looking wistful and thoughtful, Dodie began to relax. The teacher showed them how to enhance pictures instead of just cropping them. It led to even better results. Dodie walked round the display and was startled to see how much thinner she looked compared with her friends. Later, when she went home she laid out the photos. Mum admired them, "Gosh, look at you! Such an attractive young lady!" For the first time in ages, Dodie ate some dinner and didn't throw up. A text message came, inviting her to come out with a group and take photos of the area. Suddenly Dodie felt excited.

Activities

- Take photos of yourself, family or friends and try enhancing them.
- Arrange them as a montage and use to create a "makeover" show.

Materials

Cameras or phones, card, glue sticks and scissors, computer.

Discussion

- Why did Dodie stop eating? Who would you blame for this?
- Should advertisers use normal size models to sell clothes to pre-teens?
- Did you know that eating too little changes the way your brain passes messages and makes you see your mirror image as bigger than it is?
- Which foods and drinks are healthy and which ones are not?
- If a close friend showed signs of an eating problem or self-harming, how would you try to help them?
- How did comparing photos of her with her friends help Dodie?

Reflections

- Sadly, a high proportion of children, who suffer anorexia, need intensive medical support and have to be hospitalised. Tackling the issue via stories may help to prevent problems getting too entrenched.
- Bullying was the main reason Dodie stopped eating though her parents splitting up didn't help as it gave the bullies an excuse to pick on her.

- If models of average size were used to sell clothes, it might challenge the misperception of a desired perfection as essential to attractiveness. Healthy foods mean a balance of meat, vegetables, pasta, rice, beans, potatoes and fruit. Pre-packaged foods with too much salt and fat are unhealthy.

- We can try to persuade young people with anorexia to eat small portions of foods they like and will give them energy. It can encourage them to eat better, and to follow their interests and get involved in activities.

- Taking part in photography and seeing a photo of herself helped Dodie see how thin she was. It challenged her mistaken view of herself as being too fat.

- While this may seem too quick and easy a solution, this technique has been reported to be effective in work with young women suffering anorexia.

4 Social, emotional and mental health needs

Introduction: Social and emotional disability

For some children in foster, adoptive and kinship families, separations from their caregivers cause such persistent anxiety and worries that they develop phobias, obsessions, extreme shyness and panic attacks. Fears of shame, social embarrassment, difficulties with expressing feelings and with making eye contact can be painfully isolating and worsen if these problems are not addressed (Luke et al., 2014). Disability or illness may not be visible, yet inevitably raise anxiety that can feel like a paralysis. There is no "one-size-fits-all" solution to the range of problems affecting children (or parents), who have disabilities, illnesses and acute anxiety. They need someone to talk to who really understands what its like to live with their predicament. Having this support can turn what seems like a disability into strength as the young person finds their way forward.

This chapter invites exploration of how it feels to live with particular problems associated with social and emotional disabilities. The stories address selective mutism (whereby the child feels unable to speak in certain situations); autism and dyspraxia; attention deficit hyperactivity disorder; dyslexia; parental alcohol abuse; and learning difficulties. A common consequence of these issues is that affected children develop low self-esteem and an inability to believe in their potential to find their own resolutions.

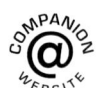

Selective mutism

Selective mutism ranges from a refusal to speak in certain situations to being socially frozen and unresponsive. Some children are selectively mute for reasons that no one knows except that they are anxious. The research presented in NHS (2019) finds no direct correlation between selective mutism and trauma or learning difficulty although these factors contribute to anxiety. Keen et al. (2008) conclude that it lies on the spectrum between shyness and severe social phobia. Anxiety prevents the selectively mute child from feeling able to speak or answer questions. Some children speak only to their family while others speak to no one. These children are not oppositional. However adults, who try to entice them to speak, may experience them as defiant, stubborn, or rejecting. Selective mutism sometimes masks more serious underlying problems. You may not know whether the anxiety belongs only to the child or to their parents.

In Story 18 Deena held her silence to protect her family to the point where her anxiety prevented her from being able to speak until Ma Domino helps her to find her voice by getting her involved in an environmental project.

How to use the story

- Invite children to engage in the activities to build their self-esteem.

- Empower the children to feel a sense of pride, value and belonging.

- Show how shyness can be overcome to gradually increase the child's confidence.

Story 18 – Deena's silence

Deena, aged 10, came from a family, who had lots of problems. Her parents had learning difficulties that made it hard for them to cope in life. They clashed and at times battered each other but told Deena not to "grass" them up. Neighbours were always reporting loud noises coming from Deena's house. As a result social workers and police officers regularly called round. Deena found it safest to say as little as possible in case she said something wrong that got them all into trouble.

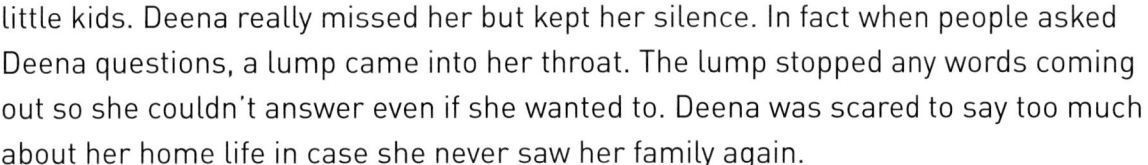

Her parents carried on having rows until Dad moved out. Deena began to miss school more often as Mum didn't get up in time to take her to school or her little sister to nursery. The school told the social worker, who visited them at home. When she saw the mess, she was so worried she took Deena to Ma Domino's. Deena's little sister was taken to another family, who had other little kids. Deena really missed her but kept her silence. In fact when people asked Deena questions, a lump came into her throat. The lump stopped any words coming out so she couldn't answer even if she wanted to. Deena was scared to say too much about her home life in case she never saw her family again.

Ma Domino was worried about Deena but not sure how to help her. Ma knew that by not speaking, Deena was missing out on such a lot. It was much harder for her to make choices about things like what she wanted to eat or drink, or activities she might like to do after school. Since Deena wasn't speaking in class it was tricky for her teacher to know if or how well she could read and what topics she had already covered in her last school. Ma Domino didn't press Deena to speak but wished she would to make life easier for herself. Instead Ma Domino showed Deena programmes on TV about causes like animal rights and environmental concerns such as with plastic waste. Deena became so interested that she interrupted the speaker protesting on the TV programme. Once Deena started speaking, it got easier. She realised she had a right to a voice and to express her opinions. Ma Domino enrolled Deena in a local environmental group. Deena began to make friends and did a presentation at school. Ma Domino told Deena how proud of her she was.

Activities

- Discuss how it must have felt for Deena to feel unable to speak.

- Dramatise scenes from the story.

- Design a poster for a cause you are interested in.

Materials

Large sizes of paper and coloured pens.

Discussion

- Why do you think Deena wasn't speaking?

- Is it hard to talk if you feel people are making judgements about you?

- What kind of help do you think children who don't talk need?

- How did her birth parents' problems affect Deena?

- Why do you think Deena found it too hard to ask to see her sister?

- What happened that prompted Deena to speak?

- What causes are you interested in?

- Would you like some help to find out more about them?

Reflections

- Young people, aged 10–14 often find it specially embarrassing to speak up when they feel they are being scrutinised and judged by others.

- Deena was frightened that if she talked she risked getting her family into trouble by giving away too much information. The less she spoke the harder it became for her to find her voice. Psychological blocks cause physical blocks like the huge lump in Deena's throat.

- The way to help someone like Deena is to be friendly and not pressurise her to speak until she feels ready, and confident enough.

- Learning difficulties make it harder for her parents to read, pay bills on time, understand written communications or meet expectations of their children's school and the authorities involved with the family. Deena's parents would have felt criticised by these people, as well as by the neighbours and been highly anxious.

- Feeling too scared to speak meant that Deena was unable to ask her caregiver or social worker if she could see her sister, whom she missed and worried about. A young person in this situation can be encouraged to draw a picture of her worries and of whom she wants to visit.

- Children, who are mute, may fear never being able to speak. The story illustrates that the process of getting involved in issues of interest and listening to speakers on these topics such as environmental concerns that Deena was drawn to can help. This can propel the child to speak up and rediscover their ability to use their voice after all.

Autism and dyspraxia

The higher functioning end of the autism continuum known as Asperger's Syndrome is now more commonly included within the more general term of autistic spectrum disorder (ASD). Affected children typically show difficulties with social aspects of communication, interaction and imagination. They also show repetitive patterns of behaviour and sensory difficulties (Wing, 1996). Symptoms such as the inability to read facial expressions, tone of voice or body language, overlap with symptoms associated with attachment disorders (Woolgar and Baldock, 2014). Many children on the autism spectrum (and children who have experienced chronic neglect) struggle to make appropriate responses or to understand other people's conversation, metaphors, jokes or sarcasm, which they interpret literally. They find it difficult to think of conversational topics, or to predict others' reactions and what might happen. They often enjoy collecting and organising items of interest to them but may hide their imagination from anyone who they sense doesn't understand them.

Autistic spectrum disorder is not linked to learning disability, but for children who have been neglected it often coincides with conditions such as dyslexia (word blindness) and dyspraxia. Dyspraxia is a neurological, developmental condition, which causes the brain to transmit inaccurate messages to the body, therein preventing the child's limbs from coordinating properly. Diagnosed in 5–6% of school-age children, four boys to every girl, dyspraxia begins early in life and slows down the ability to speak, express or explain things, or to run, throw, catch balls or skip. This also affects the child's ability in mathematics, story writing and remembering instructions. Story 19 "Dobbie's tale" describes the stress experienced by a boy diagnosed with Autism spectrum disorder and dyspraxia. Having fun in drama and creative activities helps to raise his self-esteem and improve his coordination.

How to use the story

- On reading the story, clarify that children are not to blame for their disability; the creative activities will increase capacity for self-control.

- Children who are unaccustomed to using imagination and creativity need encouragement without feeling pressurised to make eye contact.

- Invite story-making and suggest positive outcomes for their stories.

- Have children demonstrate friendly approaches using rehearsed phrases, which display an interest in others (even if they don't feel it).

- Use puppets to explain social rules and signals; rehearse changes in routine through fictional scenarios.

- Draw up timetables and plans as a memory aide, to help children feel confident of what to expect and when. If working in a group, give the affected child clear precise instructions one at a time, using visual cues, before telling the others. Invite the child to repeat the instructions but don't interrupt or the child may have to start all over again.

- Avoid ambiguous phrases the child won't relate to. Instead say, "Please lay the table" (rather than "Would you like to lay the table?")

- Involve the child in support groups such as "Asperger's United".

- Encourage willingness to learn through pursuit of special interests.

Story 19: Dobbie's tale

In Ma Domino's family, 10-year-old Dobbie was like the "double blank" in the domino pack. He often forgot things and felt he had no right to exist.

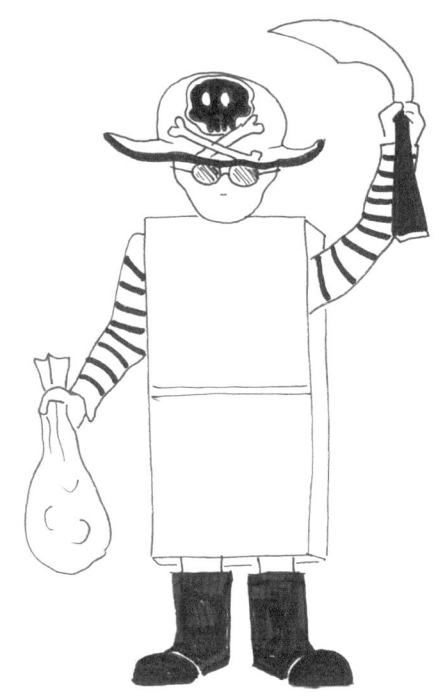

Dobbie was still a baby when his Mum disappeared from the bed & breakfast accommodation they'd been staying in. The staff found an empty whisky bottle at her bedside and a piece of paper with the phone number of Dobbie's great aunt, Dorothy. She agreed to look after him, but as he grew up, she became terribly impatient, nagging him constantly and making him feel like an idiot, no matter what he did. Dobbie could never predict her moods – she even resented him lining up his toy cars, so he kept out of her way as much as he could. One morning, Dobbie came downstairs for breakfast to find Aunt Dorothy lying on the floor. For once, she didn't shout at him, she just lay there, not moving. As it was time for school and he knew the way, Dobbie walked there and told his teachers why she hadn't come with him. By the time the ambulance reached Aunt Dorothy, she was dead. Later, Dobbie was taken to Ma Domino's. He didn't really miss his Auntie but all the changes in his routine frightened him.

Dobbie felt extremely anxious at his new school. It was bigger and a lot of clattering went on that gave him a headache. He kept going into the wrong room or bumping into someone. The worst lesson was P.E. because all his classmates could do so many more things than him. If someone threw a ball to him, Dobbie dropped it every time and had to go running after it. The teacher told him, "Pull your socks up!" Dobbie would do so, not realising she meant "try harder". He couldn't work people out. Things he said got reactions he didn't understand, like the girl crying when he asked her why she was so big. It got him the nasty nickname of "Dozy Dobbie". His teacher advised Ma Domino to take him to a specialist. Dobbie dreaded it, hating hospital smells.

At the hospital, the doctor asked questions, which Dobbie couldn't answer, just got his words all tangled up, as always happened when he felt nervous. The doctor asked him to do things like stand on one foot, then to throw and catch a ball. It was embarrassing to let her see how hard this was for him. Luckily, she was kind and said it wasn't his fault. She praised him for coping with so many changes in his life, and gave him exercises to do at home.

On the way back, they stopped at a shop that sold weird fancy dress stuff.

Ma Domino bought a pair of play swords. At home, she suggested: "Let's try out these swords like in *Pirates of the Caribbean*." Dobbie wasn't used to this kind of play. It felt strange at first but he came to really love it. Swordplay helped him concentrate. Dobbie began to make up stories and think up ideas he'd never previously had. When the other dominoes came home from school, Ma Domino invited them to play "Desert Islands". This meant making dens and building walls to keep out "intruders". Every day, Ma Domino played with Dobbie. At times when she was busy, he went on the trampoline. Jumping and somersaulting helped Dobbie get better control of his limbs. Everyone praised his efforts at trying all these new activities. For the first time ever, Dobbie began to enjoy his life.

Activities

- To help children adapt to change, invite them to walk round the room. Say, "change direction", "put one hand on your head", "touch your nose" and so on. Gradually increase the complexity of these instructions.

- Working in pairs, set up a "desert island", marking the area for a "den" with lengths of fabric and furnishing it with cushions or pillows.

- A group or family can create a "camp fire" area for "cooking" meals. Make a plan for dealing with any intruders to the camp.

- Devise a fencing routine and signals for use in "battle" to indicate when to (pretend) "die" or fall "injured" so no one gets hurt.

- Agree on a menu of favourite foods, using worksheet 5. Design invitations to a meal, using worksheet 6. Pretend to cook it.

Materials

Worksheets 5 and 6, pieces of fabric, bulldog clips, cushions, pillows, plastic swords (as protection from intruders), dressing-up clothes.

Discussion

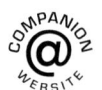

- How does being unable to run, hop or catch a ball affect a child? How long would you guess Dobbie might have had this problem?

- What is it like to be unable to read people's faces or understand them?

- Dobbie said things without realising that he was upsetting people. Can you think of tactful ways to chat without seeming nosy?

- How do you cope if someone is impatient with you? What do children need from the people looking after them?

- How does it affect a child to be told they are hopeless?

- When Dobbie saw his auntie lying on the floor what might he have thought? Was he shocked, upset, relieved? Why or why not?

- What moves and changes do you find hard? What helps?

- The teacher noticed Dobbie struggle with various movements. How does it feel to be picked out for having special needs?

- How did sword fighting, stories and drama help Dobbie? What activities would you like to try? What could happen if we wrote the next chapter?

Reflections

- Neglect from infancy increases the likelihood that a child such as Dobbie will grow up struggling to learn and feel embarrassed by this.

- Being unable to read faces or understand conversations leaves children confused and bewildered. They have to guess not only what is being said (if they don't understand the words) also, what it means.

- When a child speaks literally and upsets someone unintentionally, we can suggest ways to say things tactfully. We can explain how to use words and expressions in complementary ways. For example, when speaking of someone's large size, saying "robust" is kinder than "fat".

- Children need adults' time, patience, curiosity and willingness to listen, draw them out and involve them in something that might interest them.

- Being told you are hopeless is very damaging to self-esteem and inclines children, who lack confidence in their abilities, to stop trying.

- Seeing his Great Aunt dead might have shocked Dobbie and added to his sense of abandonment and dread of the future. Yet he might also have been relieved that she would no longer be able to bully him.

- Change is more difficult for children to manage if they feel upset and abandoned. Memory problems make it difficult to learn new routines. Pictorial timetables and maps can provide helpful prompts.

- It is embarrassing to be picked out as incompetent. On the other hand, diagnoses provide explanations and the support that the child needs.

- Creating and dramatising stories stimulates imagination and learning.

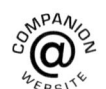

Attention deficit hyperactivity disorder (ADHD)

ADHD is the most commonly diagnosed neurodevelopmental disorder in children. It is attributed to prematurity, low birth weight and maternal smoking or alcohol use in pregnancy (Willis et al., 2017). The symptoms of post traumatic stress disorder (PTSD) are often confused with those of ADHD. Linares et al. (2005) found pre-birth absorption of drugs such as cocaine to affect children's development and behaviour. Poor sleep, hyperactivity, high energy levels, incessant chatter and raised anxiety inevitably make it difficult for the child to concentrate and learn. There is no cure and although medication can alleviate anxiety, high doses tend to have side effects of appetite suppression, drowsiness and numbness. Diagnosis has to be accurate for the medicine to be effective. Children with this condition need lots of encouragement to focus on tasks and develop skills, as well as plenty of physical exercise to use up their excess energy.

Story 20, "Drumming for Dibs" describes the experience for a boy with ADHD, who is embarrassed at being so often out of control and anticipates rejection for being in trouble until he is helped to develop skills and make friends.

How to use the story

- Read the story to discourage children from embarrassment about having ADHD. The activities that follow help to improve self-control.

- Notice which instructions or social signals the child has not understood. Give clear explanations that will assist the child in these areas.

- Encourage children to find safe ways to express their frustration.

- Remind the child to follow rules and to regard their mistakes as opportunities for learning. Run physical activities to burn energy.

Story 20: Drumming for Dibs

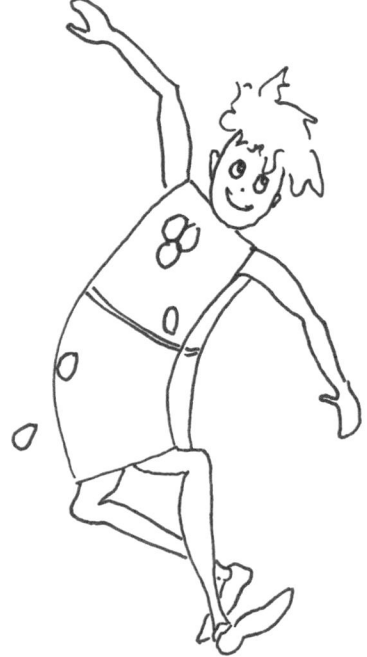

Dibs, aged 13, couldn't concentrate on anything for long. As a result of his Mum's long-term use of illegal drugs Dibs was born suffering from the effects – he cried for hours and hardly slept. Unable to cope, his Mum asked a social worker to take him away. Before Dibs came to Ma Domino's, he lived with five families, who all found him exhausting to look after. You see Dibs was constantly on the alert, expecting attack. Being perpetually on the go, he was like a spinning top or a fast running tap that no one could turn off.

As it was easy to wind him up, Dibs was often in trouble for crazy dares or fighting as doing these things made him feel alive. He made out he was "hard" and didn't care if he got told off, but Dibs was secretly scared that he was a weirdo. Sudden noises, like a door slamming made him jump out of his skin. Dibs also got scared that if he didn't eat he'd die. At meal times he tried to be first in the queue. If anyone got in his way, he elbowed, pushed, or yelled, "Go away!" which upset lots of people, While Dib's home life kept changing, treats like outings often got cancelled, leaving him disappointed, angry and left out.

But since being at Ma Domino's, Dibs was feeling calmer. Ma Domino listened in a way that convinced him he actually mattered. Noticing Dibs was often tapping his fingers, she arranged for him to have drumming lessons, in which Dibs learned to listen to the beat and follow it. His eyes shone at praise when he got it right. Before long, Dibs became keen to join the school orchestra.

At home Ma Domino sent the young dominoes to play outside but kept watch. If an argument started, she'd ask Dibs to fetch drinks and pass them round. This gave him the chance to make friends again. At times when he got carried away doing something dangerous, Ma Domino would explain why it was very important for him to be safe. She encouraged him to go off on bike rides and train himself to stop for rests, wind down and take time to think. Ma Domino read him tales about heroes and encouraged him to create his own stories. Dibs began to have better self-control and enjoy happier times.

Activities

- Make percussion instruments from junk materials:

  (a) To make shakers – fill empty jars or boxes with lentils and beans.

  (b) To make drums – have empty tins for tapping on with chopsticks.

  (c) To make a guitar – cut an oval-shaped hole in a shoebox lid and tape the lid securely on the box. Insert split pins at each end of the lid. Stretch elastic bands across the hole and round the pinheads.

- In a group, use drums and percussion instruments to express feelings. Play out "a day in your life" to illustrate the impact of arising events.

Materials

Shoeboxes, split pins, scissors, elastic bands; pulses and empty (e.g. gravy granule) containers and tins to make shakers.

Discussion

- What do you think caused Dibs' difficulties? Will a diagnosis for ADHD help him or does it risk inviting mockery and misunderstanding?

- I wonder why Dibs' Mum rejected him when he was a new baby.

- What would it be like to live in five or six foster families?

- Dibs struggled to plan ahead. Do you need help with planning?

- Dibs hated feeling like some kind of "weirdo". How did it affect him?

- What would it be like for Dibs to have to move for a sixth time?

- How did Ma Domino help Dibs? What extra help would you like?

- Do you have a favourite story? Can you tell me about it?

Reflections

- Illegal drugs taken during pregnancy affect the baby's brain and induce irritability and fidgeting. As the affected child grows up, he may run fast but struggle to concentrate and learn. Accurate diagnosis provides an explanation and access to support but there is the risk of mockery.

- Dibs' Mum had a sad and scary childhood that compelled her to put her own needs before her child's. Drugs gave her the comfort she craved. She was unable to think about how this would affect her child.

- Dib's Mum had such poor self-belief she didn't know how to make her child feel loved and secure – such patterns had never been set in her brain. She believed she wouldn't be able to give her baby the care he needed. This belief is very difficult to change without extensive and long-term skilled professional help, likely to exceed available funds.

- Such a challenging start in life makes it difficult for a child to think about his or her past or future – the child' energy tends to go into the present moment and the effort of getting from one end of the day to the other.

- Past rejection and scary memories made Dibs hyper-vigilant. Physical activities such as trampoline, football, cycling, running, Wii and gym exercises, helped to soak up his energy and enable him to feel part of the family.

- Dibs expected to have to move again as people hadn't tolerated him for long. Drumming lessons, learning social signals and making friends helped convince him that he mattered to his caregiver, Ma Domino.

Dyslexia

Dyslexia is a form of word blindness that makes it difficult to see patterns in words. Affected children will not have learned the discrete sounds of words that are mapped on to letters (Robertson and Gallant, 2019). A condition that affects many neglected children, who have rarely been spoken to, dyslexia adds to their low self-esteem, embarrassment, fear of failure and inadequacy. During the pre-teen years, the parts of the brain used to express the range of emotions develop before those applied in sensible decision-making. It is even harder for immature children, who have been neglected, to anticipate what might happen, let alone to understand other people's views. They rely on adults to help them prepare for challenging situations.

In Story 21, Den, who has dyslexia, borrows things from his brother, Dale without asking. Dale punishes him by mocking his disability. Keen on a girl, Den elicits her sympathy until witnessing the brothers' animosity she walks out. Den feels devastated while his brother gloats. Eventually, a game that requires the boys to negotiate leads them to apologise and make up.

How to use this story

- Dramatise the story to give children practice at recognition of their own and others' emotions, use their intuition, consider risks before acting impetuously, and take responsibility for rectifying their own wrongs.

- Play board games such as Diplomacy; encourage children to design board games that build the skills of negotiation and compromise.

Story 21: Den gets dumped

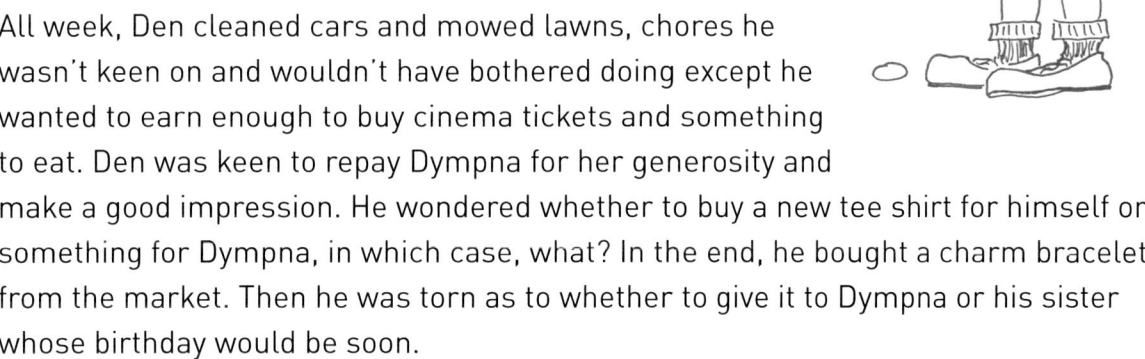

It was 14-year-old Den's first date. Last week, he'd been sitting on the ground in a games arcade, choked up with tears. Den had lost all his money and was feeling an idiot for being unable to read instructions on the machines. Dympna had passed by and stopped to ask him if he was ok, then she waited until he'd felt able to speak. Den told her he'd been about to score big time before his brother turned up and kicked the machine so hard it wouldn't pay up. Dale had laughed and run off, leaving Den broke and totally gutted. Dympna led Den to a café. She bought a burger and milkshake, and shared them. Den arranged to meet her at the same café the following Saturday evening.

All week, Den cleaned cars and mowed lawns, chores he wasn't keen on and wouldn't have bothered doing except he wanted to earn enough to buy cinema tickets and something to eat. Den was keen to repay Dympna for her generosity and make a good impression. He wondered whether to buy a new tee shirt for himself or something for Dympna, in which case, what? In the end, he bought a charm bracelet from the market. Then he was torn as to whether to give it to Dympna or his sister whose birthday would be soon.

On Saturday, Den borrowed Dale's new tee shirt but forgot to ask him if he minded. Den went to the café and met Dympna. They hadn't been there long when Dale came in with a mate and sat at the next table. Dale began talking in a loud voice about Den's dyslexia. His mate sniggered. Feeling his face turn scarlet in embarrassment Den got to his feet and decked his brother. Dale ducked and punched him back. "Stop!" shouted Dympna. Ignoring her, Den angrily snatched the ketchup and squirted it at Dale. Dympna walked out in disgust. Den rushed after her but he was too late to see where she'd gone. Upset, he stomped home and went straight to his room to avoid being quizzed on why he was home so early. The smell of fish and chips wafted upstairs. Den was hungry, but couldn't face anyone – he was too scared he'd cry.

The slam of the front door announced Dale's return. Den heard him bragging about the fight and Dympna running out. Ma Domino asked Dale to explain what happened.

Den felt guilty as he heard Dale tell her, "Dan nicked my best tee shirt and last week he 'borrowed' my game and lost it." Ma Domino called Den to come down and sent them both to the front room to apologise to each other. Neither boy wanted to but rather than be rude in front of her, they gruffly said "Sorry!" Then Ma set up a game of Monopoly. She took the role of banker and suggested they act like businessmen. As the game went on, she praised them for negotiating deals sensibly. Later, Den said he really was sorry for borrowing the shirt and promised to replace the game. Dale texted Dympna, "Sorry I spoilt your evening". Den hoped she'd still come out with him. They made plans to meet some friends and invite her along as well.

Activities

- Make up a list of your favourite songs and play the best ones.

- In pairs, print out the lyrics and decide which phrases hold the most meaning for you and why. Make up a rap or poem from these lyrics.

- In groups, play a board game such as Diplomacy or Monopoly.

Materials

Smart phone, paper, pens and crayons, board games.

Discussion

- How does dyslexia affect children? Does it affect you? How did it feel for Den to lose his money? Why do you think Dale kicked the machine?

- Den did chores to earn pocket money. Do you have to do chores at home (or school)? How can you earn money at the age of 14?

- Do you think either brother was right to feel angry with the other? Can you think of ways they could sort out their disagreements?

- How did Ma Domino help them deal with the problem?

- Do you think Dympna is likely to want to be friends with Den again? Is it a good idea for them to meet in a group? What might go wrong?

Reflections

- An inability to read makes life especially difficult for young people. It is upsetting to lose money and leaves the affected young person feeling like the world is conspiring against them.

- Dale kicked the fruit machine to get back at his brother because he was angry with him for borrowing his things and not replacing items he lost. Losing his money and being mocked upset Den.

- The brothers were both angry at each other and found it hard to back down. Talking and saying "sorry" helped.

- Ma Domino found a game through which the brothers could communicate with each other, apologise and put things right.

- An apology to Dympna might encourage her to make up with Den. Meeting in groups can help sometimes, although it can also invite the individuals to compete for attention.

Parental alcohol misuse

Noakes (2019) refers to the NHS finding that two thirds of Looked After Children have alcohol dependent parents. Many of these parents will have had poor role models for coping with frustration, their substance dependency often driven by an overwhelming sense of failure. Drink temporarily obliterates worries. The drinker feels better until the effects wear off and they feel unwell or get angry. Children of alcoholic parents may well have been exposed to unsafe acquaintances. Many will have taken responsibility for feeding themselves and their younger siblings when their parent was incapacitated. The child learns to predict the parent's mood and signs of intoxication, such as an unsteady gait, the smell on the parents' breath, a florid countenance. The child then has to calculate how best to handle things. As Coman et al. (2016) observe, children frequently blame themselves for being placed in care. Many worry that they will grow up to make the same mistakes as their parents. Some, like Dori in Story 22 use alcohol to cope. Illustrating the damaging consequences of this addiction, "Dusty's distress" features two sisters taken from their alcohol-dependent mother to live in different families. One blames the other and shows signs of alcohol addiction. The promise of help lends a degree of hope for their relationship being rebuilt.

How to use the story

- Dramatise scenes to help children realise that they were not the cause of the problem and to release themselves from self-blame.

- Help children feel proud of their ability to survive despite adversity.

Story 22: Dusty's distress

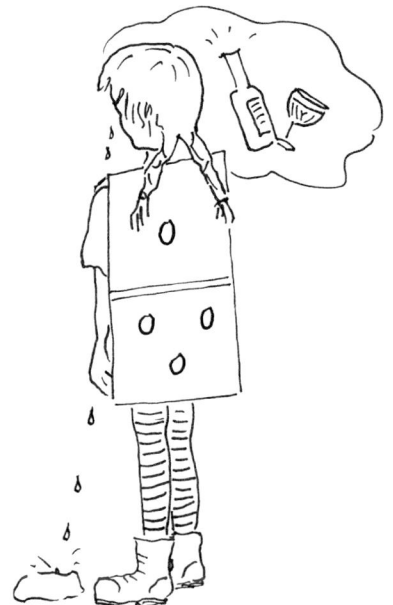

Arriving from another part of Planet Domino, Dusty, aged 13, was scared she'd never see her Mum or sister, Dori aged 12, again. This was all down to their Mum getting drunk most nights and bringing all sorts home to stay over. Some of the guys were terrifying. Dusty tried to tell someone at school but nothing came of it. Then one night, the police came to arrest Mum and bundled the girls into a car. They went on a very long journey that seemed endless. Hours later, Dusty was dropped off at Ma Dominos. As the car pulled away, she knew she'd never forget the sight of Dori's terrified face. It was the first time the sisters had been parted. Dusty felt horribly guilty and sick with anxiety. She found herself in a house with lots of young people, yet Dusty felt lost and lonely. She kept texting and phoning her Mum but got no response. Dusty knew Dori hadn't had time to find her phone when they'd left their home, so neither sister could contact the other. As time went on Dusty fretted more than ever. Eventually, Ma Domino found out where Dori was living. Dusty was very relieved to know Dori was safe. Ma Domino took her to see Dori. When they got there, Dusty was terrified to see the change in her sister. She was especially shocked as Dori turned on her shouting, "You let the police kidnap us and then you let them split us up!" Dusty cried, "No, I didn't – I had no say in it!" Dori turned her back, not listening. Her eyes looked wild as she swayed, unable to stand. None of the staff there knew how Dori had got hold of alcohol, because it was forbidden.

[From here on, apostrophes, inverted commas and bullets are not coded]Ma Domino read horrifying reports of riots on the estate the girls came from and wasn't sure how much to tell Dusty, without scaring her even more. Some weeks later, she found out that the girls' mother was in hospital with liver failure. Sadly for Dusty, it turned out to be too late. When they reached the hospital, Mum had died and they wouldn't let Dusty see the body. Ma Domino took her to the funeral. Dori was there too, but refused to speak to her. Dusty felt she'd lost everyone and everything that mattered. Afterwards, Ma Domino encouraged her to talk about her life before it was split apart. Dusty couldn't think where to start until Ma Domino prompted her. "I'm sure you have some good memories." As Dusty began to remember her life before things had got bad her eyes filled with tears. Ma Domino reassured her that these memories would give her strength to keep going and suggested, "Shall we see if Dori can live here with us – I could get someone specially trained to help you two sisters to mend your relationship." Dusty nodded, feeling a glimmer of hope.

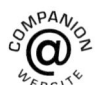

Activities

- Draw and colour in a map of the houses you've lived in – Worksheet 4.

- Write the letter from Dusty to her mother, or the letter you would like to have written to someone you miss.

- Invite your family to dramatise a scene from the story or about how differently it could have been if the girls' mother had accepted help.

Materials

Paper, size A3 and A4, crayons and pens.

Discussion

- How does being taken away from their parents feel for children?

- Can you tell if a parent has drunk too much alcohol? What can you do? Why was Dori drinking alcohol? What was she blaming Dusty for?

- Dusty was shocked and upset when Dori blamed her for everything that happened. Will it help for Dori to join Dusty at Ma Domino's? What might be the benefits? What difficulties might there be?

- If your friend drinks alcohol, what advice would you give her/him?

Reflections

- For both girls it was distressing to be separated from their Mum and each other and made them anxious. They were scared of the men, who had treated them as property. Many girls in such a situation become victims of grooming for men's gratification.

- Warning signs of drunkenness include: a swaying gait, the parent's breath smelling of alcohol, slurred words, florid face, different tone of voice and dishevelled appearance. It is not a child's responsibility to look after their parent. They should tell their teacher.

- In using alcohol for comfort, to make herself feel better Dori was emulating their Mum's way of coping.

- Dori blamed Dusty for their being parted because Dusty was a year older so she felt her sister should have been able to stop it happening.

- Ma Domino helped Dusty by taking her to visit Dori, and to the funeral. Having the opportunity to talk about what had happened should help young people in this situation, although there would be no guarantee of reconciliation.

- If Dori were to move to Ma Dominoes, provided that both girls wanted and agreed to therapeutic services, the siblings could be given psychological help to sort out their differences.

- If a friend is drinking alcohol, it is best to encourage them to seek help, by for example, telling a teacher or social worker about it so they can get some support.

Low self-esteem

Children with low self-esteem are invariably harshly self-critical and, as Sobel (2017) has noted, they continue to struggle in our UK education system. The shyest children, who find socialising a huge ordeal, may isolate themselves but still be checking and sending texts or messages to social media sites such as Snapchat and Instagram. Constant exposure to threatening posts can mean no escape for children, who are especially vulnerable. The inquiry that Jay (2013) carried out on child sexual exploitation in Rotherham found girls as young as 11 had been raped, or had witnessed rape and then been threatened that they would be next if they told. Such experiences leave the young person feeling entirely worthless. Children need adults to be vigilant, protective and interested in them. In story 23, "Daisy learns diplomacy", insult slinging initiated in self-protection led to a spiral of bullying that left the child feeling miserable and inadequate. In role-play of pre-teen problems, Daisy gains confidence on realising she knows the action needed.

How to use this story

- Read Story 23 to encourage the young people to try out methods for dealing effectively with bullying and confrontation.

- Encourage dramatic play, for practising at interpreting eye contact, voice tone, body language and when to offer and accept comfort.

- Discuss how to ensure self-protection from hostile messages.

- Discuss how much easier it is for trolls to write hostile and vicious text messages than to say these things to the person's face.

Story 23: Daisy learns diplomacy

Daisy, aged 12, did not think at all well of herself. She tried to appear confident but comments being passed around by text and various sites were upsetting her. Being called a "slag" or worse was horrible. Daisy reacted by sending insults back. The group took sides in battles that spilled over into school and usually ended in tears, Daisy often got the blame for making things worse. Her Mum had died when she was little. Daisy had since lived at Ma Domino's but had not learned how to back down from an argument. She kept wishing that she could handle things better.

One day, during break, a teacher saw Daisy getting wound up. The teacher approached Daisy and said, "Come and see me at lunchtime". Daisy was glad it was Ms Danes, whom she liked. When they met up, Ms Danes told Daisy "I was teased at school" and asked how she was feeling. Daisy admitted that the other girls had been saying mean things about her and she didn't know how to stop them. Ms Danes showed Daisy a heap of problem pages from online magazines. She said, "Let's see if we can find the answers to some of these situations. I'll be the person with a problem and you can give me advice. Pretend you're helping a mate." Daisy felt a bit self-conscious but agreed to give it a go. They looked at family conflicts, various hassles to do with texting and online messaging, and health issues such as period pains, acne and weight gain. The more they talked the more Daisy found she knew the answer to most of the problems. Role-playing gave her the confidence to take a step back and think about why people said the things they did. It helped Daisy to control her feelings and reactions and she began to feel much better.

Activities

- In pairs, practise the situations in Worksheet 7. Then swap roles to give each person a turn as the "adviser" and the "person with a problem". Then check your answers with those in the worksheet.

- In groups, make and illustrate a chart of jokey responses to put downs.

Materials

Copies of Worksheet **7** – problem pages, card and pens.

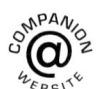

Discussion

- Why do you think Daisy didn't think well of herself? What advice would you give a mate, who gets into slanging matches?

- Can you think of characters in TV programmes such as EastEnders, who are quick to fight? What effect does this have on you? Should everyone be entitled to respect or must respect be earned?

- Cyber-bullying is increasing. How can you protect yourself? What do girls risk if they upload naked photos of themselves? Did you know it is actually illegal to post such pictures?

- How do you check on the age of someone messaging on Snapchat? Is it difficult to refuse to meet someone if they put pressure on you? What can you do to protect yourself if you decide to meet them?

- The teacher invited Daisy to "role-play" giving advice. How did this help Daisy? Can it reduce bullying? Would you like to try role-play?

- What effect does it have on bullies when their target walks away? What might happen? Can you think of any jokey responses? If Daisy wants to escape bullies, what excuse could she use?

- If all the students who wanted to stop bullying got together to confront the few individuals, who are regular bullies, the power of the group is more likely to have an effect, Can you think of ways to achieve this?

Reflections

- As a result of her Mum dying when Daisy was little she often felt unwanted if she made a fuss about things going wrong for her.

- We can encourage someone like Daisy to find out more about each person's perspective and to realise it is more effective to challenge wrong ideas by talking calmly, than insult those we don't agree with.

- Supporters of human rights promote the idea that everyone is entitled to respect. Respect is also earned by showing consideration for others.

- To avert the risk of embarrassing children, discussion of characters on TV (e.g. EastEnders), who escalate disputes, allows fictional privacy to explore ways of showing respect and consideration.

- Children need to be encouraged to delete messages and contacts of cyber-bullies and protect themselves from adults posing as teenagers on social media. Teachers need to enforce "no bullying" policies.

- The role-playing of risky situations is a way to figure out what might happen and to practise ways of handling things so you can stay safe.

- In role-play Daisy benefited from practising turning her back on a bully. Walking away can be very powerful as it disarms the bully. Practice helps young people cope in trying situations. Think of jokey responses and excuses like "I need the toilet." "I've got to meet my teacher."

- This rehearsal of threatening situations helps to deal with bullying. It may help the child to write down responses and keep the list with them. Teachers can talk about how the school can support children in preventing bullying, e.g. putting up "No Bullying" signs.

5 Difference and isolation

In our multi-racial society, the increasing proportions of ethnic minority and gay representation in politics and education reflect a broader acceptance of difference. Schools try to instil models of sharing, openness and cooperation, to give students the confidence to be who they are without infringing on others' freedom. Yet, as children and young people build their identity, they cannot help but internalise bias from the influences they encounter. Many need a strong advocate to address their anger and sense of injustice. It is always difficult to accurately deduce which factors, such as austerity, poverty, inequality, attachment, trauma, parental ill health or drug misuse, are of greatest influence on children's development. Every child and family will have reactions and responses, which are unique to them. In the interests of seeking effective ways to enable desired change it is therefore essential to keep individuality in mind, and provide more nuanced responses.

This chapter reflects on the particular experience of children aged 10–14 in adoptive, foster and kinship families, who, in addition to coping with changes of care and the loss of family relationships, are encountering intimidation, racism, sexism, homophobia and/or confusion around their gender identity. Additional issues currently manifesting in the field of child protection for some unfortunate children include the experiences of female genital mutilation and forced child marriage. The stories and discussion points are to enable children to explore predicaments through creative activities, which can help us work towards a more optimal balance.

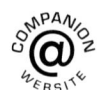

Racism

White privilege continues to be perpetuated in English schools (Bhobal, 2018). A survey from the teachers union, NASUWT, report that 37% of Black and Ethnic Minority teachers think the problem became worse in schools during 2019, noting "59% encountered every day attempts to deny the validity of their identity, thoughts, feelings or experiences – often described as micro-invalidations". As a consequence of racial bias, schools are unfairly punishing Black students for their hairstyles, wearing bandanas and "kissing teeth" (*Independent*, 21.1.20). Ofsted has observed racist language to be commonplace and most regularly expressed in name-calling. In 2014, Childline reported a rise of 69% on the previous year in calls about racist bullying, Islamophobia being the most prevalent (*Independent*, 8.1.14).

Story 24 describes the fears aroused in Donald, a Black domino, who feels too powerless to respond when challenged by a White domino to fight him. Intimidated, he backs off, and continues to be overwhelmed by anxiety until a shared smile helps him see something he has in common with another White domino and the possibility for alliances with his new classmates.

How to use the story

- Teach children about ethnicities and cultures, to encourage respect for differences as well as recognition of shared commonalities.

- Use the story and activities to explore how it feels to be a victim and why people act as they do. Encourage greater insight and empathy.

- Invite practise at walking confidently.

Story 24: Donald's story

One day, Donald, aged 11, went to school as usual. In the playground, he saw some dominoes he didn't know. They had come from another school that was being merged with his. These dominoes were white with black dots while Donald's family and friends were mostly black with white dots, although some had dyed their dots in different colours. Donald was curious. He hung around, watching and trying not to stare. A White domino came up to him, shouting, "who do you think you are c***? Wanna fight?" Donald muttered "No!" and backed away. The White guy came up closer. Donald felt really scared. Just then the bell rang and everyone had to line up to go in.

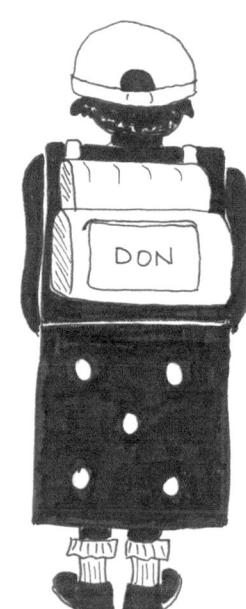

As they clattered into his classroom, Donald sat down, his heart hammering and his palms sweaty. More White dominoes arrived. The teacher announced, "Today we have some new students. I hope you'll make friends and help each other". She tried to mix the class up telling them where to sit. "Drew, sit next to Donald!" Donald recognised Drew as the one who challenged him to fight. His pulse was still racing. "Uur!" said Drew. "It's you!" He sneered at Donald.

The teacher started the lesson with a quiz. The White dominoes seemed to be calling out all the answers. Donald couldn't get anything right. He saw several of his friends on the fringes as the teacher put the class into groups, saying, "I want you all to work together!" Drew slid across to another group, so Donald began to relax and look round. He noticed some of his new classmates had coloured dots. A White domino, whose blue dots matched his, smiled at him. Donald smiled back. The White domino, pointing to Donald, asked the teacher "Can he be in our group?" Donald asked if Daisy and Dolly could come too. The teacher said they could. Suddenly, Donald realised he knew the exercise. Feeling a sense of relief he joined in and found it was more fun than usual. By the end of the lesson Donald was feeling far more confident.

Activities

• In groups of four, play a game of dominoes.

• In pairs, make two lists:

   (1) Ways in which people are the same.

   (2) Ways in which people differ to each other.

Which list is longer? Can you think of ways to celebrate the things that make us unique and that we have in common, regardless of heritage?

- In small groups, act a scene about a misunderstanding between two people. Consider how to check facts and be assertive, but tactfully. Exchange roles and repeat the scene. Discuss the arising feelings.

- In pairs (parent and child) name role models (footballers, entertainers) of varying ethnicity. Does their heritage influence their skill? Does it make it easier or harder to succeed? Or does it not affect these people at all?

Materials

A set of dominoes for each group, flipchart paper and pens.

Discussion

- How do you think Donald was feeling at the start of the story? Why did Drew challenge Donald to a fight? Was Donald right to back away? What advice would you give? Is violence ever justified?

- Was it a good idea for the dominoes to mix? Why? Or why not? How did it affect Donald? What might have helped him?

- Do you think the White dominoes were more confident or just showing off to cover their nerves? What helped Donald?

- Do you think that wearing school uniform is a good idea? Why?

Reflections

- Donald was scared to see so many White dominoes at his school and found it hard not to stare, which rattled Drew. Have you noticed how being scared causes a knot in your stomach or your throat to turn dry?

- Drew challenged Donald to a fight to prove his toughness. This was Drew's model for how to deal with conflict. Donald was probably wise to back off because violence increases anger and ill feeling. While understandable it can rarely be justified. However some people argue that wars are the only way for repressed people to get power.

- A clear anti-bullying policy for schools helps to curb racist name-calling. This can be supplemented with posters and talking through conflicts.

- The teacher's efforts to mix up the students helped Donald make a friend with a White domino and feel less anxious about mixing.

- The White dominoes may have been confident, though some are likely to be just as anxious as Donald and his friends were. However White people are less likely to encounter daily racism than people of colour.

- When Donald saw something that he and a White domino had in common, this encouraged him to make friends.

- School uniform has the benefit of being a visible sign of membership of the school. It saves children from wondering what to wear to school. Disadvantages are the insistence of some schools to homogenise everyone and disallow the distinctive styles of particular cultures.

- Teachers can help their students to feel more confident by inviting their opinions and giving them support to express themselves, provided the expression of their opinions doesn't infringe too unfairly on others.

Intimidation

It is important that we try to educate children to be inclusive and show positive attitudes, especially in the light of the threat to human rights in the UK since the vote to leave the European Union (Heald et al., 2018). The task of influencing those who are most resistant to inclusion requires understanding the underlying reason for their resistance. Some children are inclined to interpret any unintended bump as "deliberate". Even people with fixed views may be more open to influence if they sense their perceptions are validated as rational in the context of their experience. Adults can help by listening and conveying belief in children's ability to absorb multiple views and make useful contributions on living harmoniously. Story 25 illustrates some of the fears behind racist attitudes. Drew's family is materially poor and resent any they see as better off and more socially competent. Their sense of injustice drives them to take revenge. This story illustrates how influences of kindness and friendship bring change.

How to use the story

- Dramatise the story to explore why Drew's family acted as they did.

- Discuss ways in which children of varying ethnicity can share thoughts and debate differing viewpoints safely without fear of being bullied.

- Discuss how "culture" may be distinguished from "race".

- Give the children practice at challenging discriminatory attitudes, by remarking, "I wish you didn't say those things. Please stop."

- Uphold policies on protection from racism and bullying.

Story 25: Drew's dare

Drew, an 11-year-old White domino, had grown up
hating lots of people, especially Blacks, who looked
posh. His family scorned anyone they saw as different.
Their home was like a tatty box, grubby and worn out
from rough handling.

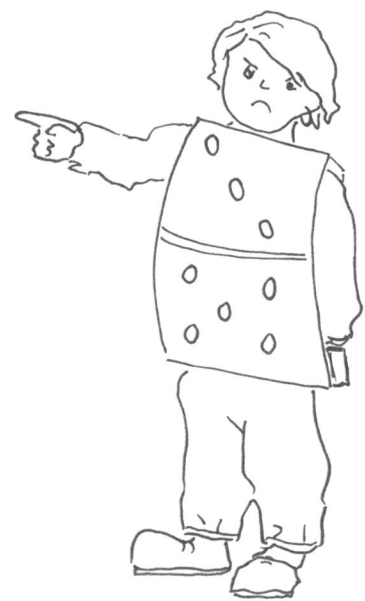

It was Drew's first day at his new school. When he got
there he was put out to see lots of Black dominoes
looking smart and slick. It made him feel dumb,
pathetic, somehow. If any of them looked his way, he
would challenge them to a fight to prove he wasn't
scared. It gave him a thrill, a sense of power. When he
got home, Drew announced that his school was now full
of Black dominos. His Dad said, "It's not right, them getting an education an' their
parents taking jobs off us an all!" Nodding agreement, his uncle said "It's totally out
of order – we'll show 'em what's what!" Their aggressiveness and glint in their eyes
left Drew nervous.

One night soon after that, his family went out taking a truckload of muck with them.
They watched some Black dominoes gliding into a smart, tidy house. A short time
later, Drew's family poured the muck through the letterbox of that house but got
caught. Later that night, the police took Drew and his sister, Destiny, to Ma Domino's.
Drew was scared and angry at being taken away. He fumed, "I'll make them Blacks
pay for this! If it weren't for them, this would never have happened!" Destiny sneered,
"Bet you ain't got the bottle! Go on, trash the school, I dare you!" She didn't mean it
but he took her seriously.

A few days later, Drew sneaked out and set off in the direction of his school. Destiny
heard him leave and followed him. It was raining hard and already the school
driveway was under water. Drew vaulted over the gate, but landed awkwardly and
hurt his arm. Destiny clambered up behind and fell on top of him. Donald, a Black
domino, was leaving his drama club when he heard Destiny yell. He ran across
asking "Are you ok? Can you move?" Destiny nodded so he helped her get up. Donald
guessed Drew had been planning to do something he shouldn't. He phoned Ma
Domino for a lift home for all three of them then told Drew, "Don't worry, I'll say you
came to meet me." Drew was amazed! He'd rarely met such kindness. "Thanks" he
said, gruffly.

Later when they were warm and dry, Donald told Drew about the Drama club. "Quite a few of our class go. It's a blast, man – seriously, you should try it! We're doing stuff about gangs. Reckon you'd be great at the stunts!" Drew told him he'd never been to any clubs, as his parents couldn't afford them. Donald asked Ma Domino if Drew could go to Drama Club and she agreed to find out. Drew wasn't too sure but once he got there they rehearsed fighting scenes. It turned out to be exhausting but they had a lot of laughs. The boys started hanging out, finding more in common than Drew would have guessed. In fact having a mate was proving ok, far less scary now, and teachers had stopped picking on him so much. Drew was sad that his parents were in prison but he felt safer at Ma Domino's, where he found it so much easier to have mates.

Activities

- In small groups, improvise a scene from the differing viewpoints of Drew, Donald and the teacher. Show each scene to the large group.

- In pairs, practise dealing with racism, then share ideas with the group.

Discussion

- Why did Drew hate anyone who looked different from him? How do we typecast people? Can we influence those with views we disagree with?

- What made Drew think the Black dominoes were smarter than him?

- If you felt left out or bullied, what would help you to feel included?

- Why do you think Destiny dared Drew to trash the school? How did Donald help? What do Drew and Donald have in common?

Reflections

- Drew had grown up in a family that held fixed, stereotypical racist views. For example they believed that immigrants had stolen their jobs and housing so they shouldn't be allowed to stay. It is extremely difficult to change such fixed views.

- Journalists have a responsibility to make known relevant statistics that challenge certain racist assertions. We all have responsibility to treat people with the quality of respect we want to receive ourselves.

- Drew noticed the Black dominoes looked shinier and in better shape than him. Lacking self-belief, his assumption that they knew more and learned faster than him made him envious and jealous.

- Drew was influenced by his family's resentment of Blacks, whose presence in his school gave his family the excuse to take out their anger on them.

- By having more youth provision and mixed schools, we can influence people to have more accurate perceptions and understanding. We can value cultural differences without making it a cause for fear, dispute and jealousy.

- Drew's sister's daring him to trash the school was rooted in a desire to goad him. She wanted to make something happen that would get her brother into trouble.

- Donald's invitation to the drama club helped him and Drew forge a new friendship. Having fun changed Drew's attitude. It helped both young people to enjoy things they had in common.

Gender and homophobia

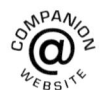

Roles around gender identity shape behaviour and the way others perceive us (Winfield, 2019). Most pre-pubescent children prefer the company of their own gender, but as they approach adolescence, many start to experience anxiety around gender identity. A young person who prefers their own gender comes to fear being seen as "weird", or "gay" – a word frequently used as an insult, albeit adopted by the homosexual community. While equal opportunity laws have made it easier for gay people to marry and hold positions of power, hostile name-calling arouses fear of bullying and social exclusion. Some young people choose to be referred to using the gender-neutral pronoun "they" – rather than "he" or "she" (Newman and Newman, 2018), which allows them to pick a non-binary pronoun that reflects their identity and feels right for them. At age 10–14, the importance of peer acceptance makes it difficult to take up interests seen to be the province of the opposite gender. Children depend on adults to support them in the right to choose their identity and develop their personality and skills. Reflecting on prejudice rooted in fear, "Dami's disgust" is about two girls whose friendship gets sabotaged.

How to use the story

- Use Story 26 to reflect on the importance of mutual trust and respect.

- Dramatise a scene in which the word "gay" is used as an insult; give the children practice at responding appropriately to nasty jibes.

- Parents and teachers can encourage celebration and understanding of all identities within lessons, assemblies etc. (and educating others).

- Discuss how both genders could be encouraged to try out and benefit from special interest areas such as mechanics and dance.

Story 26: Dami's disgust

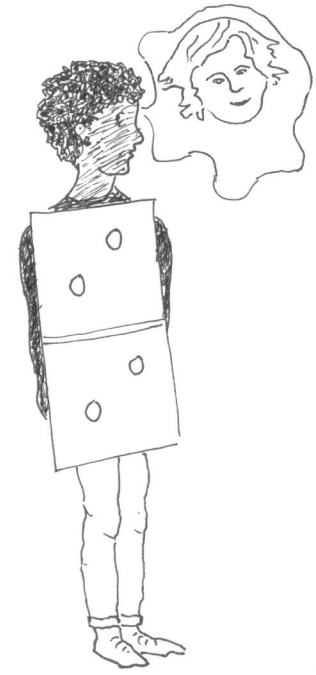

Dami, aged 12, is adopted. Her parents encourage her to be proud of herself but their edges are rounded, whereas Dami's are squared off. Being Black, Dami often feels "different" from her schoolmates. Even so, having recently visited the town she came from, she is relieved to have been adopted.

At her school there are dominoes of various shape and colour, which Dami reckons is cool. They all mix in and get on, so Dami didn't expect any hassle from being best mates with Dizzy, a White domino. Dami felt huge warmth for Dizzy. They'd got to know each other in an action group trying to get publicity to keep a family safe from threats of deportation. After a few of these meetings, Dami and Dizzy started to look for somewhere more private to hang out together. They found an allotment shed. Here, safe from prying eyes, they chatted about everything and shared secrets as they swapped things like games and hairbands. Dami was really happy, but Dizzy was nervous in case someone found out and told her Dad about her friend. He was so old-fashioned in his views she knew instinctively that he wouldn't approve of Dami.

One evening, a neighbour saw the girls going into the shed, holding hands. "How sweet!" she thought and told Dizzy's Dad about it, unaware of how he'd react. Dizzy's Dad was appalled and disgusted. He grounded Dizzy and made her promise to have nothing more to do with Dami. In school the next day, Dami kept trying to catch her friend's eye but Dizzy looked away and at break she disappeared. On the way home, Dami caught her up. Dizzy refused to meet her eyes but told Dami they couldn't meet up anymore because her Dad had forbidden it. Since her Mum had left, he'd got very strict and she couldn't risk disobeying him. Dami was devastated. Hearing of the things Dizzy's Dad had said made her feel something was wrong with her. Dami was blinded by tears and stumbled into another classmate, who asked her why she was upset. Dusty took her to Ma Domino's, where she was living. Dusty and Ma Domino were so kind that Dami felt ok to tell them what had happened. She moaned, "I can't work out why Dizzy is being like this! I mean, why should it be a problem for us to be close friends?" Ma Domino remarked that friendship was very important. She explained that some people believe it is unnatural and wrong to allow people of the same gender to kiss let alone have a sexual relationship. These views are wrong but people who hold them frown on any openly affectionate behaviour. Ma emphasised that this view only incites fear and bigotry.

Disgusted, Dami said, "That's insane!" Ma Domino agreed. "Yes, such a wall takes a long time to break down." Dusty said, "It's so unfair not being allowed to be close with the friend you get on best with." Dami reckoned everyone she knew in her class preferred to be with their own gender, at least some of the time. This led to another debate. Dami knew many of the boys were mad on sport while the girls preferred shopping, doing their nails and stuff. Ma Domino said "It would help if schools tried harder to get more girls into sports and sciences and more boys into the subject areas geared mainly to girls." Dusty felt better, now that she felt she understood some of the arguments.

Activities

- Draw pictures of the characters in this story, on card and cut them out.

- In small groups, act the scene, in which Dizzy gets home from the allotment. Decide how the other classmates will react the next day.

- Write a poem about friendship, using Worksheet 8 as a template.

- On Worksheet 9, draw things you'd like to keep in your shed.

- In pairs, make a list of "causes" popularly supported by 10–14 year olds e.g. environmental issues, fair trading, animal rights etc.

- Design a poster for a cause and state why you think it's important.

- In groups/pairs make a list of activities adopted by mostly one gender and decide how the other gender could be persuaded to try them out.

Materials

Flip chart, A4 paper, pens and crayons, copies of Worksheets 8 and 9.

Discussion

- Dami felt different from the rest of her family. Do you think being adopted affected her? How might looking different affect you? If the shade of dots matched feelings, what colours might yours be? What helps children to sense they belong with their friends/family?

- Dami and Dizzy joined an action group for protecting people from deportation. Are you interested in this or any other social issues?

- Why do you think Dizzy's Dad stopped her friendship with Dami? Can you guess what he said? How does it make you feel? How might you try to persuade Dizzy's Dad to soften his sharp edges?

- How would you feel if a close mate ended your friendship? Why might Dami think there was something wrong with her? At what age do most children start thinking about gender identity?

- Do you think having to wear school uniform might help or hinder Dami? What helps young people to be more accepting of each other?

- Would you try a new activity or subject if it was mostly being taken up by the opposite gender? Would a drama or filmmaking group appeal?

- What could Dami's next adventure be? Shall we write/draw it?

Reflections

- While most grow up to be attracted to the opposite sex, some children have a strong physical and emotional attraction to the same gender. They may be wary of showing their feelings, and scared of how they'll be treated.

- Being adopted can also contribute to feeling "different" especially if the child's ethnicity and appearance are noticeably different to that of their family. Being stared at can make adoptees feel very exposed.

- Adoptive parents can help their children feel they belong by talking to them about their experiences and reassuring them of their love.

- At ages 10–14, many children become interested in causes and social issues, such as animal welfare, deportation and environmental concerns such as carbon footprints and plastic waste etc.

- Dizzy's Dad showed racial and gender prejudice and intolerance. The school could invite him in and challenge his ideas about these issues. Dami was hurt and disappointed by Dizzy's rejection of her. Being told it was wrong to love a girl made Dami feel something was wrong with her. Ages 10–14 years is the time when children think about gender identity.

- Hairstyles e.g. big hair and headwear (scarves etc.) can be annoying for teachers trying to maintain rules. Having hard-to-tame hair could place Dami at risk of criticism. Schools need to be culturally sensitive to this and model tolerance.

- Girls can be encouraged to take up football, woodwork, sciences, and boys to take up dance, drama, home economics, childcare etc.

Sexism – the right to respect

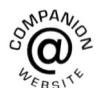

Undermining the right to respect is a prevailing culture that objectifies women and encourages teenage boys to view girls as commodities (like dolls) whose feelings are irrelevant (Zimbardo and Colombe, 2012). Dines (2011) found boys from the age of 11 surfing porn, as much out of their need for information as for salacious interest. To win peer approval, some teenage boys boast of sexual conquests and show lack of understanding about mutual consent. Sales (2016) remarks that girls as young as 12 are cajoled or bullied into sex before they are ready. Many are convinced that they must do what is asked of them if they want to hold on to their boyfriend, avoid rejection and the anonymity of having no partner. This is especially concerning for girls in care or adopted, whose experience of rejection may leave them so desperate for acceptance and a sense of belonging that they comply to avert rejection.

Illustrating that respect for others emerges from self-respect, Story 27 "Derry and Des" features twin boys, whose experience of neglect and abuse left them with poor social skills until they learn to relate more sensitively to girls.

How to use the story

- Discuss the sources of disrespectful attitudes and behaviour.

- Explain why the minimum legal age for sex is 16+.

- Dramatise the story to show why the law is needed to protect them.

- Give the children practice in saying "no" to unwelcome coercion.

- Talk about the effects of porn; explore how to navigate relationships.

- Compare the effects of welcome and unwelcome remarks.

Story 27: Derry and Des

Derry and Des were twin brothers, aged 13, who had been
thrown out of their last home. Ma Domino was asked to look after
them and drove over to pick them up from the hostel. As they
got into her car, the twins started laughing manically. She asked
"What's the joke?" They laughed even harder in a higher pitch.
Politely, she asked them to be quieter because the traffic was
busy. Rudely, Des replied, "Why? Have you only just passed your
test?" and Derry laughed even louder. Ma Domino began to feel
so stressed that when the traffic lights turned green, she stalled
the car for the first time in years. The brothers nearly split their
sides. "Told you she can't drive! She's a f ***g woman after all!"
Ma Domino clenched her teeth, tempted to tell them to get out,
but resolved to drive home and see what she could do about it.
It was Friday night, so she knew it would be difficult to arrange
for her new guests to stay anywhere else over the weekend, but
already she was worried about how they'd behave with her girls.
When she showed the twins their room, they demanded money.
Ma Domino said it was out of the question for now. She explained: "In this house we
treat people with respect. When you show respect, you will get privileges like pocket
money but not until then."

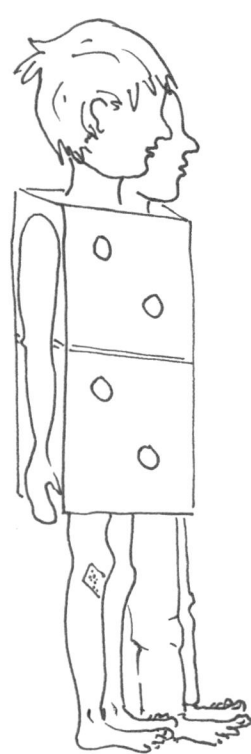

Ma Domino was always polite and friendly. After a while Derry and Des tried to copy
the manners she demonstrated but they often forgot. Their father's violence meant
they had never felt safe. Their mother had always told them not to make a fuss and
didn't seem bothered by their Dad's cruelty to them. Hurt by her lack of concern, the
twins didn't recognise their own feelings let alone anyone else's. Lately they had been
playing online fantasy games that featured girls as dolls you could do anything you
liked with. Derry and Des made sexist remarks that embarrassed the Domino girls.
They realised the twins didn't actually know the meaning of what they were saying, or
how to get on with people. Ma Domino tried to explain to the twins why their language
was so demeaning and offensive but she didn't get very far. The girls decided to try
and teach Derry and Des to show respect. They drew cartoons of boys talking to girls.
In speech bubbles, the girls wrote "dos" and "don'ts". They explained what "respect"
meant and encouraged the twins to practise showing it by chatting in a friendly, polite
manner. To keep a safe eye on things, Ma Domino hung around, bringing drinks and
crisps. As the girls spent time with the twins and were patient with them, Derry and

139

Des began to feel more confident and welcome in this home so made more efforts to impress them.

Activities

- Draw cartoon figures of girls and boys, using Worksheet 10.

- Make a list of compliments that a boy or girl might welcome.

- With your parent or sibling, practise making these compliments, and notice the effect they have.

- List unpleasant remarks in common use. Discuss why such remarks are used, even when they are not welcome.

Materials

Large sheets of paper and felt tip pens.

Discussion

- How did the twins' manic laughter affect Ma Domino? What effect did their sneering at girls and women have?

- As soon as they came to Ma Domino's, the twins asked for money. Do you think Ma Domino's response was reasonable or a bit unfair?

- What kind of manners do you think she wanted them to show? Is it hard for teenage boys to talk to girls? What is respect? What (if any) remarks on their appearance should girls tolerate?

Reflections

- The twins' manic laughter and demeaning remarks rattled Ma Domino, affecting her ability to think clearly and concentrate on driving.

- The twins had grown up learning to deride girls and women. Their birth parents had sneered at talk of feelings and the idea of caring about appearances, both of which they regarded as weaknesses.

- The twins felt betrayed by their Mum's casual dismissal of their Dad's cruelty and her failure to protect them. This destroyed their trust in her.

- The twins were acting much younger than their age. Ma Domino needed to respond to this sensitively but firmly. Her boundaries kept the twins and her girls safe. She expected the twins to be polite, show respect, wait their turn and make an effort to get on with people.

- Teenage boys, who are not used to girls, can become crippled with shyness. Some cover this up with bravado, showing off to raise laughs without realising the effect that mockery and derision can have.

- It is important for responsible adults to model attitudes of kindness, empathy, interest, respect, and to stand up to bullies.

- If a person makes unwelcome comments we can ask them to leave the room and only come back when they are ready to be sociable.

- It may be necessary to explain to the young person why their comments are so unwelcome and suggest things to say instead.

- Respect is about showing due regard for feelings, wishes and rights of others, admiration for another's abilities, qualities or achievements. Girls should only respond to remarks on their appearance if the comments are complimentary and evidently well intentioned.

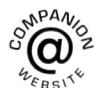

Female genital mutilation

Female genital mutilation (FGM), also known as "cutting" or "circumcision", is a procedure carried out on girls and young women of all ages from infancy on. FGM involves removing all or part of the external genitals for non-medical reasons. Not all survive the procedure due to loss of blood, infection and not receiving medical attention. Von Rege and Campion (2017) remark that FGM has no health benefits and carries a high risk of physical and psychological harm. In the UK, it has been officially banned since 2015, where involved professionals are mandated to report known cases to the police. Yet as a deeply entrenched, centuries old cultural practice, FGM continues to be carried out in secret in over 30 countries, mainly Africa, but also parts of India and the Middle East. It is regarded as a "rite of passage" and an important part of the child's identity to ensure purity before marriage. The belief is that a girl who has been cut will be good and make her family proud. If not cut, she will think about sex, turn into a slut, thereby bring shame on the family and no man will marry her.

The shame runs so deep that the girls are taught never to touch or look at their genitals. Many, who are cut in infancy, only find out when they attempt to have sex. They then have to be cut again to consummate a marriage and again when they give birth. Reconstructive surgery can restore some of the missing parts but FGM frequently causes irreversible damage. A problem in the UK is that the safeguarding measures of repeated questioning can be seen as discriminatory. Dixon et al. (2019) remark that it risks being counter-productive if it discourages use of services. Story 28 illustrates a child's experience of FGM and goes on to describe how she was helped to cope with her disturbing memories and the changes in her life that followed.

How to use this story

- Read the story and talk about feelings experienced by its characters.

- Look at a map of the world and identify where the countries are.

- Discuss what cultural practices should be respected and which not.

- Explain the importance of telling someone if you don't feel safe.

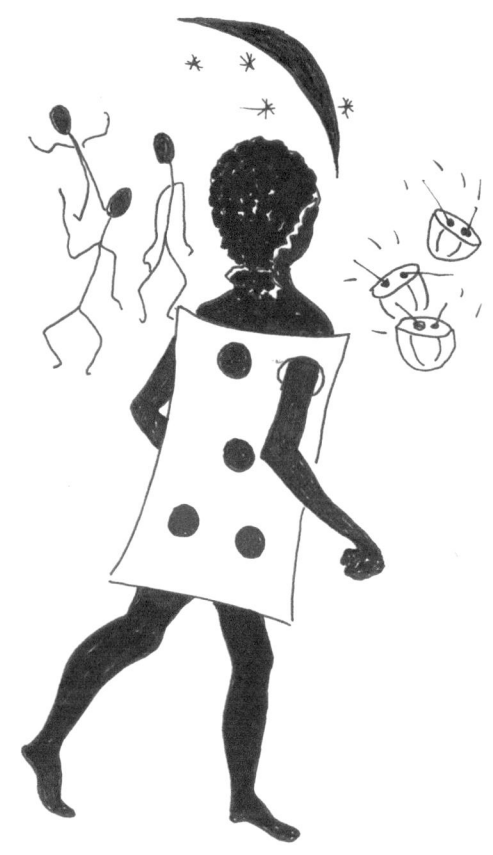

Story 28: Dukha's secret

Dukha, aged 10, came to Planet Domino from another part of the world, where her life had been very different. She had a painful secret she was trying hard to forget. It hurt very much but the trouble was she couldn't tell anyone, not even kindly Ma Domino as it felt way too embarrassing and shaming.

It happened a few months ago in the place she'd lived all her life before coming to Ma Domino's. On her 10th birthday Dukha's Mum had sent her and her friends to a party down by the river, near the woods. When they arrived, several girls and boys were there already. Drums had been set up and tables were loaded with food that smelled delicious. Dukha felt excited. There was lots of singing and dancing and treats being handed round. They were having such a lovely time until suddenly Dukha noticed one girl after another being led off. Most of the girls had gone when Dukha and her best mate heard ear-splitting screams from the woods. Terrified, they bolted but the boys chased after them and half dragged half carried them back to the woods, where the other girls were crying. One of the older women told Dukha, "You're next!" She and three others pinned Dukha down then plunged a knife into the most painful place possible and ripped her apart, before sewing her up. The pain was so terrible that Dukha passed out. She woke up to find her legs tied together, making it impossible for her to go to the toilet.

Dukha was carted back to her Mum but could hardly bear to speak to her. She cried, "How could you let them do this to me?" Her Mum told her. "Its to make sure you will make us proud of you! If you don't have it, no man will want to marry you!" Dukha said, "I never want to marry if this is what I have to put up with!" Her Dad was working away but when he received Dukha's letter, he came home and put her on a plane to Planet Domino. Dukha was taken to Ma Domino's but she didn't feel safe and still suffered the most agonising pain.

One day at school, Dukha was in too much pain to do PE. The teacher phoned Ma Domino, who came to collect her and was surprised that Dukha refused to see a

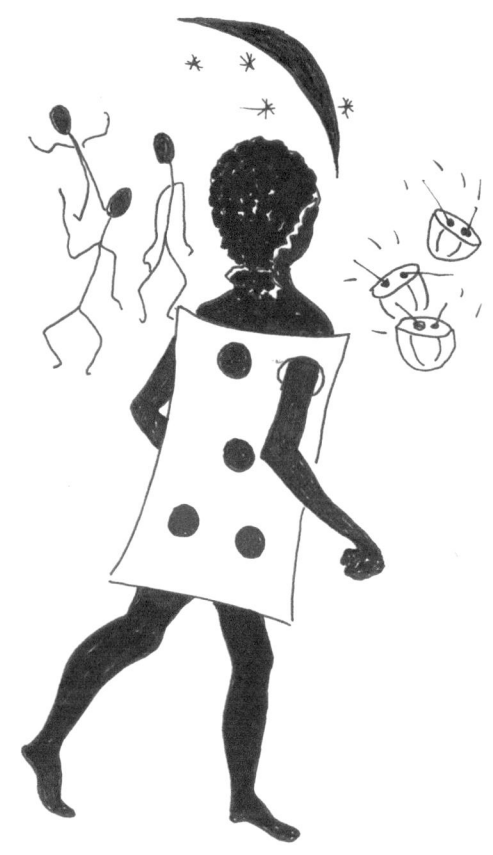

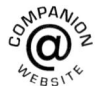

doctor. She heard Dukha crying in the bathroom and asked her what was upsetting her so much but Dukha couldn't explain.

Guessing what Dukha had been through Ma Domino told her a story about a young bear, who lost his tummy button. His cruel parent bears had burned it, leaving a hole that was thankfully masked by the fur growing around it. The young bear was rescued and came to realise that life was possible without his tummy button. Still, he knew it wasn't there and he was angry with his parents for their cruelty. He wanted to know why they did it and what he'd done to deserve it. Dukha burst into tears again, but now she felt brave enough to explain the pain she was experiencing. Ma Domino listened with tears in her eyes. She said, "You've been so brave, but now when you feel safe enough you must start telling your story – it's not healthy to keep it locked away."

Activities

- Develop the story about the bear by drawing it as a cartoon.

- Decide which country Dukha came from. Look up stories from it.

- Play recordings of music from that country.

- With drums and percussion instruments hold a "concert of feelings".

- Choose a postcard of a scene that makes you feel peaceful. Place it in the centre of A4 paper. Using crayons or paint, expand the picture on the postcard to fill the paper round it. Remove the card, fill in the gap and identify which part you most like. When you feel stressed, count to 10 and think back to being in this peaceful place

Materials

Scenic postcards, pastels, crayons, pens and paper, tablet for looking up information; music player or phone, drums, percussion instruments.

Discussion

- How do you think the bear felt about losing his tummy button?

- Why do you think some parents are so very cruel to their children?

- Can you think of any cultural traditions that are good fun to follow?

- Are there ways to stop harmful practices? How can we try to influence people? By making laws or just talking about it?

- How might a painful experience affect you when you grow up?

Reflections

- Losing part of himself left the young bear feeling different. A human being in such a situation is also likely to feel isolated and lonely.

- Parents may be too caught up with their own needs, to think about the effects of their actions on their children. Cultural rules can prompt parents to feel compelled to fit in and obey rules, in order to avoid disapproval and being cast out by their family and community.

- Parents might also fear for their child's future if they don't follow these rules. In some cases, when parents have experienced too little love and care in childhood they become cruel in response to a child crying. The parent mistakenly assumes their child hates them and is deliberately trying to upset them.

- There are plenty of fun, enriching cultural traditions such as festivals, religions, music, methods of cooking and eating particular foods, dressing in costumes unique to their culture, which provide valued support.

- Adults should always try to avoid inflicting pain on a child without good reason. Arguably an exception to this rule is vaccinations, which protect children from the spread of disease. In contrast, the pain caused by FGM is hideous and permanently damaging.

- There are various ways to bring about change via legal means and to influence people. This can be achieved through social meetings, health clinics, home visits and clubs. It is important to share feelings and stories about FGM. Posters giving facts and statistics can be displayed, for example in GP waiting rooms and school reception areas etc.

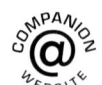

Forced child marriage

The World Health Organisation (WHO) and Inter-Parliamentary Union's report (Scolaro et al., 2016, p. 4) describe forced child marriage as a "human rights violation that robs a girl of her childhood". Forced child marriage disrupts their education and social development. It also endangers health and growth and increases their risk of exposure to violence and abuse. While practised mainly in the Asia-Pacific regions, it is widespread elsewhere in Eastern Europe and in America, where fourteen states still allow 13-year-old girls to marry (Gray, 2020). In 2015 the Human Rights Council voted to end child forced marriage. Internationally, there is agreement to the minimum age for marriage being 18 years. Yet barriers to implementing effective protective measures continue to exist.

Girls and women are allotted a lower social status in patriarchal structures, which enable men and boys to assume rights over girls' futures. Poverty is one of the reasons that in parts of India and Africa, girls as young as 8 years 9 months are sold into marriage, often as a convenient solution to settling debts. Marrying off children is also a long-standing cultural safeguard against premarital sex and immoral acts. Save the Children (2016) estimate that "One girl under 15 is married every seven seconds". This includes girls as young as 10 in Afghanistan, Yemen, India and Somalia. UNICEF (2018) also estimate that in addition to over 650 million women alive today being married before the age of 18, in 2016, another 5.6 million girls under 18 became child brides, some giving birth to their first child before the age of 15. These young women are therefore deprived of their opportunity to attend school or further education or the right to be free of slavery. Women in that situation become vulnerable to domestic abuse, being forced into sex and contracting diseases such as HIV.

Story 29, "Dilip and Drina's drama" illustrates the powerlessness of young Dilip, forced into marriage at the age of 13. Her sister, Drina, is rescued but lives in constant anxiety about what is happening to Dilip.

How to use this story

- Read Story 29. Find out how many countries in the world allow the forced marriage of children to be practised.

- Discuss the reasons for its continuation.

- Why do you think these countries allow forced marriage?

- How can these attitudes and traditions be changed?
- Talk about what governments and local authorities should be doing.
- How can a young person check on the age and identity of someone who is contacting her on Snapchat, pretending to be her age?

Story 29: Drina and Dilip's drama

Drina arrived at Ma Domino's after an organiser of a women's campaign to protect children from slavery wrote to Ma Domino and put Drina on a plane to Planet Domino, where she'd be safer. Ma Domino went to the airport to collect Drina and bring her to the Domino home. The organisation was still trying to rescue Drina's sister Dilip, who, at 12 years old, had been sold into marriage.

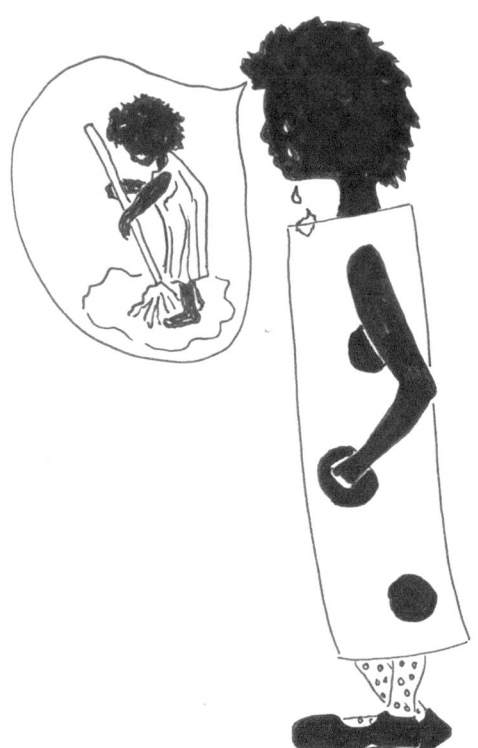

A few months before this happened the girls' parents were killed because their Dad hadn't agreed with the army's politics. Dilip and Drina ran away, knowing they had no choice or they too would be killed. After weeks of searching for shelter and scavenging for food anywhere they could find it, the girls met a friendly man, who offered them food from his stall and seemed really kind. After promising to look after them, he led them to his house. Several other girls were living there too. Dilip and Drina were grateful that at least now they would be safe and could get to school. But within a few weeks the man sold Dilip to someone, who was willing to pay him money for her. Dilip had to leave school and from then on she spent her days sweeping the floor, washing dishes and clothes, collecting firewood and cooking her husband's dinner in the evening. He bullied and whipped her if she didn't do everything he demanded.

Drina tried to find out where her sister was but that turned out to be a closely guarded secret. One day a woman came to the school to give a talk. She was representing the organisation trying to protect girls from being sold into marriage. On their way out of school Drina told the speaker about Dilip. The woman arranged for Drina to go to Planet Domino, where Drina soon realised that forced marriage wasn't practised. She was relieved to be safe but even more worried about her sister, who was yet to be found and rescued.

Ma Domino tried to answer Drina's questions about why her sister had been sold. As they talked about forced marriage, the other dominoes were horrified and said they would tell everyone they knew, to try and get Dilip rescued.

Activities

- Read the story. Decide which part of it you would like to focus on and how you would like the story to turn out.

- Using junk materials, make a model of the landscape for the story.

- Draw the main characters, stick them to card and cut them out to use for dramatising the story.

- Dramatise scenes in which Dilip's husband controls her and prevents her from expressing her views or using her knowledge.

- Outline a map of parts of the world where forced marriage is practised.

- Arrange a discussion of this issue at school.

Materials

Maps of the world, large pieces of paper (A1 or A2), A4 paper, felt tips, paints, scissors, PVA glue, junk materials – boxes, scrunched paper, kitchen roll etc.

Discussion

- How can you tell if an adult you depend on can be trusted?

- Talk about the separate experiences for Dilip and Drina.

- How do you think each sister felt about her ordeal?

- How does it affect you if or when you are forced to do things that you consider are unfair or wrong?

- Discuss ways in which children should be protected from harm.

- Talk about how else we can influence people to change.

Reflections

- It is always hard to tell if people are trustworthy until you know them. Dilip and Drina felt they had little choice but to follow the man, who promised shelter. He then took money in exchange for Dilip, who was enslaved against her will. Trust is built on knowing you can depend on someone to deliver promises, turn up on time, be reliable, friendly etc.

- Both girls had lost their parents and escaped from the war in their home country to avoid being killed. Being hungry they were forced to scavenge for food. They became exhausted and had sore feet.

- For Dilip, being forced into marriage at 12 was abusive. She lost her freedom, education and any chance of fulfilling her ambitions. Dilip would have felt crushed, abused, betrayed, hurt and very angry.

- Drina was fortunately rescued but lives with the anxiety of what is happening to her sister and devastated on her behalf, possibly also feeling guilty for having escaped the same fate.

- Trauma makes the brain hyper alert to anticipated dangers. It would leave a girl such as Dilip feeling perpetually fearful, depressed and hopeless. As trauma has a deleterious effect on concentration Drina would find it harder to learn, access educational opportunities or make trusting relationships even in a comparatively safe environment.

- Laws imposing duties on responsible adults to report missing children are helping to raise the profile of children at risk of forced marriage.

- If you suspect this is happening to a girl in your class, it is important to tell a teacher. Instances of forced marriage have reduced but there is a long way to go. Support groups can also help protect girls at risk.

6 Social media pressures

The last decade has seen a steady rise in the use of social media, which has the undoubted benefits of connecting people across the world and has proved immensely useful during the lockdown to limit the spread of the Coronavirus. Even so social media has increasingly been shown to have many detrimental effects on children's well-being: interrupted sleep patterns, anxiety about body image, "sexting", grooming, cyber-bullying, screen and game addiction, also, radicalisation. A UK government report (House of Commons Science and Technology Committee, 2019) finds 70% of 12–15-year-olds to have a profile on social media and 12.8% of children aged 10–15 years to be spending more than three hours on social networking on a normal school day. Screen time is displacing healthier activities such as physical exercise, face-to-face socialising or reading a book. The increase of social media pressures has led to rising mental ill health. The report identified three areas of concern:

Content – what material the children are looking at.

Contact – who they are talking to – such as adults, using fabricated identities.

Conduct – how they conduct themselves, e.g. online bullies and victims.

This chapter addresses issues of cyber-bullying, gang-related crime, the fear of missing out driven by advertising and peer pressure, online game addiction, idealisation and anxiety about body image, and children's access to porn. The stories illustrate predicaments for the young person and how involved adults can utilise dramatic play and creative activities as a means for talking through the impact and encouraging the children's interest in healthier pursuits.

Cyber-bullying

In today's society, multiple social and media influences are increasingly being reinforced by peer pressure through cyber-bullying. This occurs in a variety of settings and typically includes harassment, humiliation, insults and/or threats (Festi and Quandt, 2017). The most vulnerable children, whose identity is already fragile, are often desperate for peer approval and fear rejection. For pre-adolescents, the dread of being unable to meet expectations, to own the latest technological products and be up to speed with on-line gossip affects their self-esteem. When these pressures are added to stressors associated with having to cope with changes of care, difficulties in meeting academic expectations and conflict in relationships, encounters with cyber-bullying has induced post-traumatic stress symptoms especially for girls (Baldry et al., 2018). It has also led to self-harming behaviour (see "Self-harm", Chapter 2). Parents and caregivers can support children by preparing them in advance for likely challenges. Story 30 "Decision for Dana" focuses on the power exerted by peer influence and illustrates the young person using her wits to extricate herself from trouble and deciding to choose her friends more carefully in future.

How to use the story

- Read the story and use the creative activities to explore related topics.

- Reflect on the importance of valuing friends for their personality, rather than for their looks, possessions or clothes.

- Through discussing the pros and cons of social networking, guide the children to delete malicious messages and report the senders.

Story 30: Decision for Dana

Dana, aged 14, had recently come to Ma Domino's after her Mum walked out and her Dad decided he could no longer cope. Some girls at her last school knew her family had split up. They said cruel things like that her Mum only left because Dana was too greedy and demanding. Dana had started to believe the many nasty text messages telling her she was ugly, selfish and stupid. She despised herself and had almost stopped eating more than the tiniest morsels. Dana believed she was fat, though by now she was very thin and actually hated the sight and texture of food. In fact, even the smell of cooking sickened her.

What Dana wanted most of all was to have friends and be part of a group and she dreaded going to her new school. It was the middle of the term so she expected everyone else to have someone to sit with. She feared getting bullied. During class on the first day at her new school, Dana got a text inviting her to meet up later. When the teacher wasn't looking her way, Dana saw the girl who sent it looking at her and nodded back thrilled to be chosen. At lunchtime, she found out that this girl was in a gang of White dominoes, who said they were going out that night "looking for action". They were planning to graffiti the place of some Blacks they hated and insisted, "you're coming with us". Dana was nervous. She badly wanted friends and at least this lot seemed up for a laugh. Very persuasively, they swore it would be "amazing" but Dana was scared of getting into trouble and knew it was wrong to pick on people. Bravely she said, "I'm not sure I'm cool with that". When they got back to class, a text message came, warning her not to grass because if she did, her life would be unliveable – "We know all about you!" – it said. So Dana decided she'd better keep in with them for now. She tried to get out of it by fibbing that she'd lost her phone, but they told her to nick one. That was just the start of it. At home she saw a phone lying around and on impulse she picked it up. It was Dudley's phone and he was extremely upset when he couldn't find it. Dana texted the girl who'd invited her then told Ma she'd be studying at a friend's house. Unusually, Ma Domino was too busy with another crisis to check her story. At dinnertime, Dana was feeling so stressed she even forgot how much she hated baked potato until a bit got stuck in her throat. Her face turned bright red as she choked. Everyone stared and Dana wished the floor would open to swallow her up. Being praised for eating made her feel even worse, knowing that Ma would not like what she was getting herself into.

Dana had just left the house when the phone buzzed with a message telling her where to meet the gang. She'd tried excuses like "I'm not allowed" but it hadn't worked as they'd given her an alibi. Walking to meet them, Dana saw the gang already starting to spray the walls of a house. Someone inside the house was crying. Dana's stomach churned. Feeling sick rise in her throat she went behind a fence to throw up. The gang was laughing as they sprayed racist insults, but weren't looking her way so Dana saw her chance and ran. Tearing down a passage between houses, she bumped into a police officer who asked her, 'Where are you off to?' Pointing to the house being spray-painted, she legged it as the officer radio'd for help. The gang was arrested and charged. Luckily, no one suspected Dana. From then on Dana was more careful about choosing her friends. She gave Dudley his phone back and avoided troublemakers. Ma Domino asked her to help with jobs. Sensing Fate had given her another chance Dana began eating again.

Activities

- Think of messages to combat bullying and racism. Spray them onto large pieces of card (size A1 or A2).

- Draw the story's characters onto A4 card and colour them in. Cut them out and make a small stand for each character.

- With your family, act out scenes from the story. Set a scene in court and talk about how racism and bullying could or should be dealt with.

- Practise what you might say to a bully, "No! I'm not going to do that!"

Materials

White card size A1 or A2 and A4; spray paint, crayons and pens.

Discussion

- Why do you think Dana stopped eating? What might have helped her? Some children develop eating problems due to fear of looking fat. How important is it to have a figure that pleases other people? Who do you think influences 10-14s the most – their friends, parents or advertisers?

- Do you find cyber bullying a problem? How can young people protect themselves from this? What effect does bullying have? How can we stop it? Do you think more CCTV (at school or shops) is a good idea?

- If a child has to change school mid-term what would help her/him?

- Why do children join gangs? Do you know anyone who has to obey their gang's rules? Why do you think the White gang picked on Black people? Dana felt under pressure to join in the gang's activity. What else could she have done? Should she have told a teacher about the gang's plans?

- Dana took Dudley's phone. How did that affect him? Have you ever had things stolen from you? How did it make you feel?

- Why was Dana embarrassed when she was being praised for eating?

- Dana's stomach churned when she heard the person crying inside the house. Can you think of places to escape to if necessary? When and where have you seen racism? How can it be stopped?

Reflections

- Dana gave up eating because she believed the nasty text messages. Her Mum should have been more aware of Dana's distress and eating too little. Talking about the effect of parents' separation helps. Having to move school meant Dana had lost her friendship networks. When moving school mid-term children will be helped to adjust if they visit the new school in advance and once in their new school are enabled to visit their old school and stay in touch with friends, say in recreation groups or perhaps via social media, or a phone call etc.

- A child who has stopped eating because of stress can be reassured she is not as overweight as she thinks and encouraged to eat small helpings. Beat is an organisation that provides advice and support for young people who have eating problems.

- Parents, friends and media all have an influence. No child can avoid being influenced by their parents, who are their main role models for how to manage life. At 10–14, friends become an important influence. Adverts influence us subliminally. The widely available perfect images of models serve to convince us of the need to aim for this perfection.

- Everyone wants friends. Gangs are a means of achieving membership of a group when there are no alternatives such as sport or youth clubs.

- Cyber-bullying has a very bad effect on the recipient's self-esteem and confidence. It is all too easy (especially if they've already experienced rejection) to believe the nasty things said by bullies. Children can learn strategies for dealing with bullying, including reporting it.

- In the story the gang targeting Black people is an example of racist abuse. Dana could have told a teacher or Ma Domino about it.

- Dana felt embarrassed and a bit guilty about deceiving Ma Domino. When she heard the victim crying Dana felt so bad, she ran off, no longer willing to be part of making things worse. She knew it would be important to make a stand against racism and not get drawn into it.

Gang-related crime

Social media, advertising, music, films and online games communicate the vital importance of money. Yet for many young people whose parents are hard up, money is inaccessible. Cuts in youth services in the UK have left young people without safe places to "hang out". A recent study of 91 adolescents explored the conduct and emotional problems of gang youth and non-gang youth (Wood, 2020). Gang-related youth were found to have higher levels of conduct disorder and exposure to violence than non-gang youth. The need for money is a prime motivator for gang-related violence including knife crime. This violence leads to seriously detrimental outcomes for already deprived communities. The media have reported on gangs recruiting children as young as 11 into drug crime and using them as "drug mules" in county line trading to distribute drugs (Andel, 2019), a scenario illustrated in Story 31. Another approach to changing young people's fear-induced perceptions, and make communities safer, is suggested by Gilbert and Sinclair (2019) who demonstrate the effectiveness of showing films on the effects of gang violence to children at school and discussing the facts about knife crime with the students.

How to use this story

- Read the story and invite the young person to draw or dramatise it.

- Explain the facts of knife crime – i.e. it is illegal to carry any object that could be used as a weapon without a good reason for it.

- Discuss the effects of knife crime on the victims, bystanders, family and the community where they live, also on the perpetrator.

Story 31: Dean escapes the "No's"

It was freezing cold outside. Dean, aged 13, shivered in the narrow stairwell, waiting for a signal. His uncle, Diego, had demanded a favour he couldn't refuse. You see, since his parents died, Dean was living with Diego and had nowhere else to go. The favour was to pass on packages of brown stuff. Diego said it was a business that was going to make them rich but it hadn't happened yet. In his uncle's gang, "The No's", Dean had watched some girls smash up the brown stuff and sort it into packages that he was to deliver. Diego reckoned the police were less likely to pick on Dean, who was small for his age. Dean felt for the knife hidden inside his jeans. Having it made him feel safer and gave him a bit of street cred. As a member of Diego's gang, Dean found it necessary to earn respect by doing things like being rude to teachers, stealing stuff and robbing people, which won him extra points.

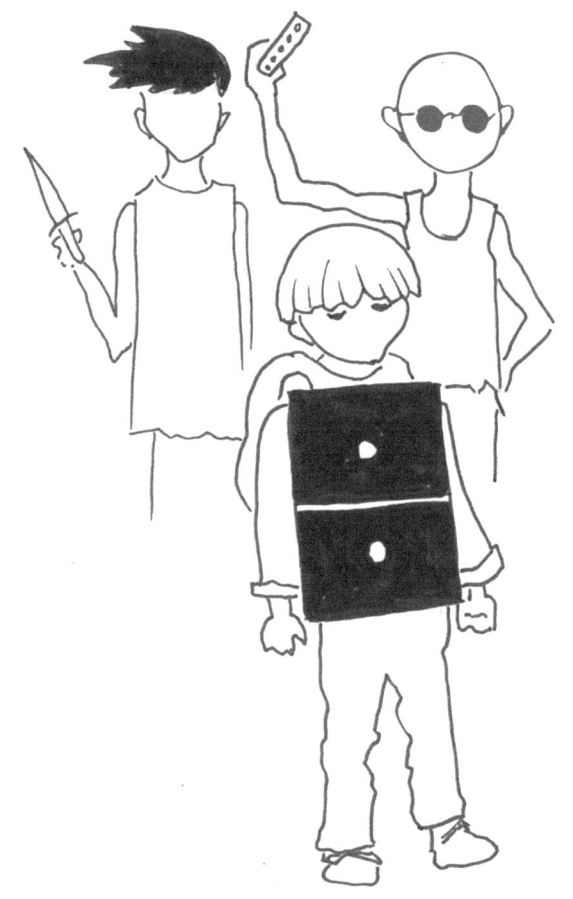

All of a sudden Dean heard sirens and saw police cars racing into the close. The officers got out and tried to surround the gang. One of the officers collared Diego, who spun round, stabbed her then ran away, yelling at Dean to run too. Seeing blood pouring all over the ground Dean felt sick with horror. His blood rushed to his ears as he raced off as fast as he could. He kept running but the police seemed to know all the places to hide and soon caught him. Dean wound up at Ma Domino's place, where he learned that carrying weapons and acting hard wasn't the best way to go about things. Ma Domino involved him in various sports that got him enthused and meeting others like him. Dean was very relieved not to be in prison for carrying a weapon.

Activities

- Act the scene in which Diego asks Dean to deliver packages of drugs.

- Have a player beat a drum to convey emotions as the scene unfolds.

- Find out about the laws and legal penalties for knife crime.
- Create a scene in court where the judge decides on Dean's future.
- Draw the characters and show who gets their spots rubbed off.

Materials

Drums (or saucepan to drum on), drumsticks, judge's wig (optional).

Discussion

- Why do you think Dean got involved in Diego's gang? How did it affect him? Did showing a tough front require gang members to look hard and sharp at the edges? Who does knife and gun crime affect and how?

- Why do you think Dean was carrying a knife? Did it make him safer? Have you ever tried carrying a weapon with you? Was it any help?

- Do you know what the legal penalty is if caught for carrying a knife? What could be the sentence if someone dies from a knife attack?

- Which jobs entitle you to carry a knife? If you were not going to or from work, do you still have an excuse to have a work knife on you?

- At what age can shops sell knives and cutlery to young people?

- What future opportunities can knife crime affect the assailant?

Reflections

- Dean became a member of Diego's gang while he was living with his uncle after his parents died. Dean believed he could not refuse to go along with Diego. He felt he had no choice.

- Although carrying a knife made Dean feel safer, this is a myth since the research shows it is more likely to lead to further violence and people getting hurt.

- The sentence for carrying a knife can be up to four years in prison. If someone dies from a knife wound, the attacker can be sentenced for life.

- Jobs such as carpet cutting and kitchen fitting entitle you to carry a knife to and from your place of work. If you are not going to work or coming home from it, you are not entitled to carry any kind of offensive weapon.

- You have to be 18 years old to purchase a knife legally.

- Knife and gun crime affects victims, their families, and their communities. Its effects are invariably devastating and long lasting.

- The future opportunities that affect knife crime assailants include being barred from admission to college or university.

- You will also be barred from other countries, including the USA, Canada, Australia and New Zealand.

- A criminal record for knife crime severely curtails job prospects.

Fear of missing out

From the age of 10, children generally want to belong to a peer group. Social media and the ability to see through a rose-tinted lens what everyone is up to amplifies the sense that lots of events are happening to which the young person has not been invited. Media power exerts so much pressure (Twenge, 2017) that the young person becomes anxious about what he is missing out on. It isn't possible to be everywhere at all times and often what is seen and heard on social media is an idealistic snapshot rather than the reality of the event. Desire for things that will make them feel good and meet their friends' approval motivates some to obtain goods in any way they can in order to feel accepted. Some children in care will have been trained by their poverty stricken, disenfranchised parents to steal. Their parents may be illiterate and therefore unregistered or unable to access any help, or they may be illegal immigrants or hiding from the police. The most neglected children may not realise or understand the moral implications of theft. In Story 32 the yearning to look "cool" prompts Dan to steal a coveted iPhone. The humiliation of being caught plunges him into shame until a new friend helps him learn about trust.

How to use the story

- In pairs (or small groups) dramatise scenes from the story, to help the young people recognise that actions have consequences.

- Encourage them to view mistakes as experiments and opportunities to learn rather than as shameful evidence of inadequacy or immorality.

- Young people can use the fictional role to practise ways to say "sorry", forgive and make recompense for their mistakes.

- Talk about how to avert traps that could lead you into trouble. Invite the young people to enjoy new friendships from shared interests.

Story 32: Dan's dare

Dan, aged 11, was feeling bored and left out. He arrived in Ma Domino's family a few months ago but though she tried to make him feel wanted, he often felt he didn't deserve to exist. The trouble was Dan didn't have nearly enough loving care when he was little. His parents were in prison and Dan sensed that he, too, was bad. He did things that got him into trouble and people didn't include him in their groups. Dan was lonely and wished he could be like his popular classmates who seemed to get to all the parties and have tons more stuff than him. It felt so unfair! One day, Dan wandered into a Tech shop and spotted an iPhone – the very model he most wanted. He knew people got away with nicking things and he thought, "I really need that phone!" Then he figured "They won't notice if one of them goes missing." The shop was busy, so Dan took a chance and quickly stuffed the phone inside his jacket. But as he slipped outside, the shop alarm went off. The cashier yelled, "Hey you! Come back here!" Scared, Dan ran home. Before long, the manager phoned Ma Domino and told her Dan had been seen taking the phone and was banned. Ma promised he'd return the phone. As the manager knew her, he agreed not to tell the police.

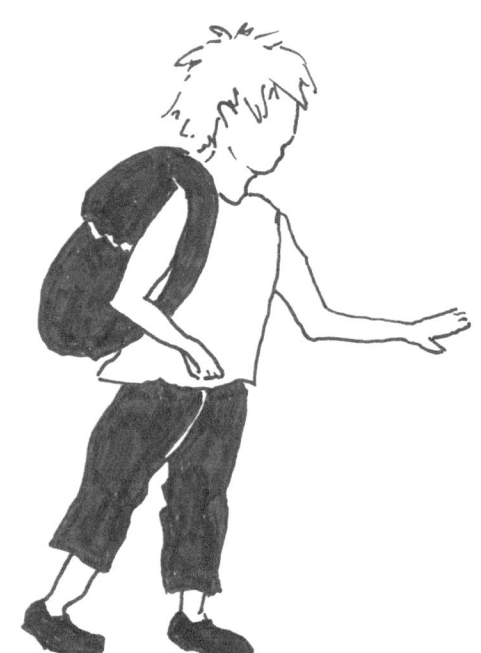

Ma Domino asked Dan why he'd taken the phone, but he didn't reply. He just kept wondering why she was making such a big deal of it. After all his real Mum and Dad wouldn't have cared. In any case, Dan was sure she'd never understand why it was so important for him to have it. Ma told him, "You're banned from that shop." Dan replied, "I don't care!" This was his usual reply when he was in trouble. But deep down, he hated upsetting her. It was just too uncool, embarrassing, to admit to, that's all. In fact, Ma Domino knew that Dan was only pretending he didn't care and was actually quite lonely. She grounded him but a few days later he was looking so unhappy, she suggested he ask his mate round. Unfortunately his mate's Mum had heard about what happened in the shop and wouldn't let him come. Embarrassed, Ma Domino was now even more worried. Then she had an idea and invited her nephew, Dray, round instead.

Dan found Dray friendly and easy to talk to. Dan soon took Dray to his room and got out his computer games. They discovered they liked the same music and both loved the FIFA game. At dinner, Ma Domino asked Dray what he wanted in a friend. Dray said, "Someone you can trust and depend on" and added "I like Dan because he's a laugh and shares his stuff." After tea, the boys went into the garden for a kick around. "I'll show you the park" said Dan. On the way, they passed the shop he was banned from. Dray wanted to look inside. Dan explained why he wasn't allowed in. Listening sympathetically, Dray said "Yeah that happens to loads of people. Practically everyone tries to get away with nicking something at least once. It's FOMO isn't it? You know – fear of missing out. There's so much we all want and can't have. Anyway, everyone makes mistakes, that's how you learn, isn't it!" Shrugging, miserably Dan said, "Trouble is, everyone at school hates me now! Even my best mate won't speak to me." Dray said, "Try not to worry! When people find out they can trust you, they'll forget what happened. Share your games and you'll soon have mates again." They started chatting about levels they'd reached and swapped games. Dan took Dray's advice and found people friendlier when he showed interest and asked them about things they liked talking about. From then on, he proved he could be trusted – well mostly.

Activities

- Design a strip for the football team (or other sport).
- Make a poster of items you'd like to have. Add photos of friends and family, food you like, favourite places and pictures of your interests.
- Find out about part-time jobs where people your age can earn money.
- Enact the scene between Dan and Dray, to practise friendship skills.

Materials

Card, crayons, magazines, glue sticks, scissors, felt tips, photos.

Discussion

- At the start of the story, Dan felt bored and left out. Can you think of activities he could be doing? What activities might you enjoy?
- Why did Dan believe no one cared about him? Who can you go to if you need advice or support? What help do you need at home/school?

- What makes young people want to break rules? Which rules do you think are fair or unfair? Are there any rules that are/aren't necessary?

- Did Dan have a good reason for stealing the phone from the shop? Do you think the ban was fair? How could he put things right?

- Dan's classmate wasn't allowed to visit him. Was this fair? How should parents protect a child from someone they think isn't a good influence?

- How do you think Dan felt when Dray wanted to go in the phone shop?

- Dray thinks trust between friends is essential. How can you tell if someone is trustworthy? What qualities are important?

- If your friends found out that you'd taken something of theirs, how long do you think it would take them to trust you again?

- What do you think of Dray's advice?

- What interests do you share with your friends, or would like to?

Reflections

- When Dan was feeling bored, he could have looked for a game to play or someone to kick a ball around with, or tried, say, junk modelling.

- Dan felt no one cared about him because his parents had given him too little attention. Consequently he didn't know how to amuse himself and wouldn't think of finding an activity when he was bored.

- Children in school may need an adult to go to when they feel anxious. They may regard certain rules as unfair, particularly if they are enforced for students but not teachers (like being allowed to use a particular short cut, or go indoors when its raining or use the library at break time). Some rules (timetables) are essential for safety and consistency.

- The shop manager had to impose a ban, to protect his business and avoid Dan and other children taking too much advantage.

- At first Dan couldn't see that what he'd done was so wrong and thought Ma Domino was making too big a deal of it. Dan's belief that he should be able to steal things if other people got away with it came partly from his parents and grandparents, who had regularly stolen.

- Dan's closest classmate wasn't allowed to visit him. His mate's Mum wanted to protect her son from wrong influences. Was this reasonable?

- Dray helped Dan to learn about trust – the importance of sharing things and keeping your word as a friend. Dan realised he wanted to be trusted. He decided from then on he wasn't going to steal any more.

- When trust is broken it takes a long time to mend. If you are aware that you might breach trust and take your friends for granted it helps to buy time to think first. Sharing interests also helps to build friendship.

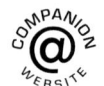

On-line game addiction

Technology stretches minds but also entices children to spend excessive time on their phones and games. Chat rooms enable virtual contact with lots of people but this allows far less time to communicate directly and read faces. Screen addiction is affecting the emotional circuitry of children's brains, which depend on face-to-face interaction to learn non-verbal signals. Compounding the problem is the more violent content of on-line games in which actions have no consequence and has led to a decline in young people's empathy (Zimbardo and Coloumbe, 2012). West et al. (2017) discovered that playing these games reduced grey matter in the hippocampus, unless the player uses strategies of navigation to enhance it. This addiction is also leading to health problems of inadequate fresh air and poor sleep for the young players.

Demonstrating that success builds on itself, Story 33 "Dariel's obsession" illustrates the dangers of game addiction, which result in reduced sleep and poor grades. The story shows how a new friend encourages the young person to try new face-to-face activities and consequently enjoy much better health.

How to use the story

- Use the discussion points to talk about the impact of online gaming.

- Invite the children to practise reading non-verbal signals.

- Show pictures of different facial expressions and what they reveal.

- Use the suggested creative activities to encourage children to talk to their friends face-to-face, not just via texting or chat rooms.

Story 33: Dariel's obsession

Dariel, aged 12, loved computer games – Star Wars, FIFA, especially the latest games and any that were rated 15+ or even 18+. Dariel played these games every day after school until late into the night and took on any willing opponent. The buzz it gave him made up for the tedium of school where he was slipping further and further behind. Lack of sleep and exercise was leaving him too exhausted to concentrate and last the school day.

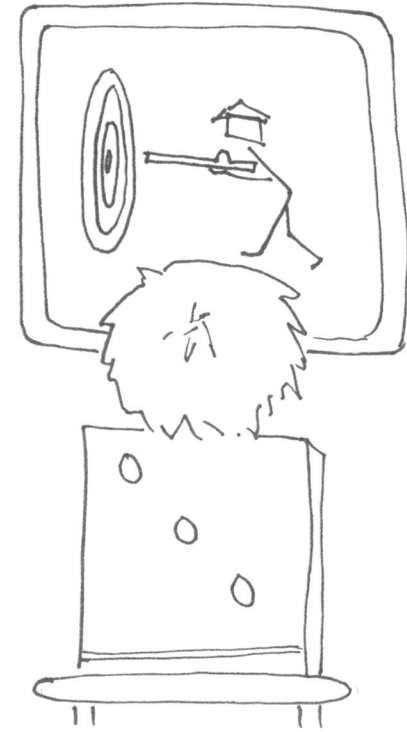

Dariel was shy so it suited him to be alone in his room where he didn't need to be sociable. But he'd become obsessed with games and being interrupted while he was playing them made him so wild, he'd swear at whoever did it. Ma Domino noticed Dariel looking pale and being rude and irritable when she asked him to do anything. To get him some exercise and social opportunities, she sent him on an activity holiday where he had to join in team events like assault courses, cycling, canoeing, pony trekking, swimming and climbing. It was a wet spring and Dariel hated getting soaked and muddy. He couldn't bear these sorts of activities. It didn't help that his arms and legs were now growing fast and making him clumsy. Jeering from the other guys made him feel a total loser and as far as girls were concerned, like he didn't even exist. He couldn't wait to get back to online games but Ma Domino was in despair.

Near the end of the summer term, Sports Day arrived. It was raining, so the sports teacher decided to hold it indoors. He set up Wii, skittles, darts, and old-fashioned table games like dominoes, draughts, chess and cards. Dariel played chess with Dorrie. She beat him but he didn't mind because the way she rolled her eyes made him smile. He found her easy to talk to and she laughed when he did. Seeing everyone enjoying the activities gave the sports teacher an idea. He came over to Dorrie and Dariel and asked them if they'd like to help him set up an indoor games club. Looking at Dariel, Dorrie said, "Yeah, sure, I'm up for it, if you are?" Dariel found himself agreeing to help.

Organising activities for the club left him far less time to play on-line games. In fact, now that he was getting on so well with Dorrie, playing games by himself was no longer quite as much fun. Dariel was enjoying the social side of the club more than he'd ever dreamed of. Once he realised he was just as good at these games as his computer games it felt great to be part of a group. He enjoyed the admiration of the others in his class, who noticed he was ok at most games. At times he still craved the thrill of violence in games like "Tomb Raider", but as invitations kept coming, Dariel's confidence grew. All the exercise and fresh air meant he was sleeping well and feeling better.

Activities

- The young person and parent draw domino characters and paste them onto card; divide into pieces and number as follows: Head – 1, arms – 2 and 3; legs 4, and 5 and Body – 6.

- Roll the dice and when it lands on a six start by selecting the body of your character. Throw a "one" to place the head on the body and so on. The first player to assemble their cartoon figure wins the game.

- Make a list of alternative words to use instead of swear words.

- Practise ways to ask a friend if they'd like to play or do an activity with you, and ways to ask a group if you can join in their game.

Materials

Crayons, paper, magazines, glue sticks, scissors and dice.

Discussion

- Why did Dariel become so keen to play on-line games?

- What was their main appeal? Which games do you like?

- What are the drawbacks of game addiction? What helps you recover?

- How does it feel to lack social confidence?

- What led Dariel to try out social activities he'd previously avoided?

Reflections

- Playing online games gave Dariel a convenient way out of socialising. He was very shy and often struggled to think of smart things to say.

- Dariel found online games far more exciting than school or homework.

- He got high scores and games didn't make impossible demands.

- Playing these games late into the night meant Dariel was getting too little sleep so he was too tired to concentrate in school, and his marks suffered. He became irritable and rude if he was interrupted while playing. How does playing computer games affect you?

- Getting no exercise and fresh air was bad for Dariel's health.

- We can help children recover from this addiction by encouraging them to try new activities, exercise, social events, and to get enough sleep.

- When children lack confidence in social situations, they can be encouraged to make one friend at a time to begin with. This will take the pressure off the child to manage group situations. The friend can help the child to feel valued and important.

- The combination of making friends with Dorrie, and finding he was enjoying different kinds of games including being involved in forming a club led Dariel to try out social activities that he'd previously avoided.

Idealisation

The media – Internet, films, television, advertisements, hoardings – saturate us with images of toned, slim bodies. These images entice girls and young women to believe that something is wrong with them if they don't have the ideal look or shape even though such airbrushed perfection is unattainable in reality. Research finds that to stay slim, one in four children aged 10 years skip meals and one in ten at this age are "extremely worried" about becoming fat (Carey, 2016, 149). NHS statistics found that a third of children aged 2–15 years to be overweight and under exercising (*Independent* 22.8.13). Around 11–14 years is an age of acute self-consciousness (Blakemore, 2018) when lack of confidence and fear of ridicule are huge obstacles to taking up exercise. It is even harder for girls, who constantly worry about rejection, having grown up to believe they will never be able to live up to desired perfection. Story 34 illustrates the value of exercise for enhancing emotional health and life skills. Desiré is afraid she is too fat to dance but after being upset by a rival, she is encouraged to realise her talent, so worries less and enjoys dancing.

How to use the story

- Explain that the motivation behind denigration is to take power over someone, and is a form of bullying.

- Use the creative activity to explore messages elicited from the way girls and women dress and present themselves.

- Encourage the child to keep a diary, to enhance her self-knowledge.

- Provide a dance mat, Wii dance routine, or invite the child to create one, to encourage relaxation and enjoyment of physical activity.

Story 34: Dancing for Desiré

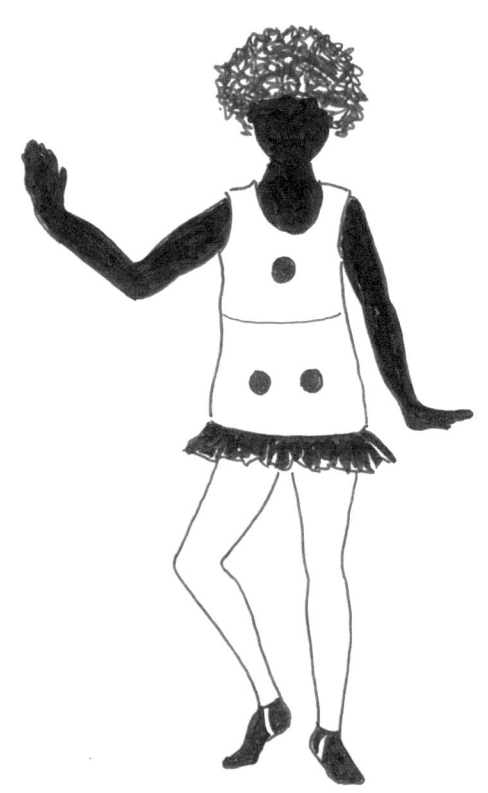

Desiré, aged 12, was keen to live up to her name. Ma Domino told her it meant she was beautiful, but Desiré didn't believe it. Her parents died a few years ago. She still missed them and wished she could ask them if it was true. Desiré was generously built and growing in every direction. Her clothes were getting too short and tight. The skinny, perfect, models on TV and in online fashion images made her scared she was getting way too fat. The boys in her class had started calling her "Fatso", which upset her. Ma Domino overheard her telling a friend about it on the phone. Ma suggested "How about joining a dance class? You're such a great mover, you'd love it!" Desiré said, "Nah, everyone who goes to those things is skinny. They'd laugh at me! I'd look ridiculous!" Ma Domino, who was also generously built, asked, "Is that how you think I look?" Desiré said "No of course not! But…". So Ma Domino rang a friend whose daughter went to the dance class that was nearest.

The next day, Suzy came round and persuaded Desiré to come to the class. Desiré loved dancing and was enjoying herself until she heard someone behind her sniggering. Turning round, she asked, "Is there a problem?" A skinny girl said rudely, "Yeah! I can't see anything when I'm behind you, your bum's blocking my view and you're doing it all wrong. It's putting me off!" Desiré felt crushed. Her eyes welled up and she felt a massive lump in her throat. She ran to the toilets and locked the door, then daren't come out in case anyone saw her crying. Suzy came and pleaded with her to go back. "You've got to! Ms Davenport thinks you're brilliant! You don't want to listen to that stupid girl – she's only jealous because you're a better dancer than her!"

Desiré let Suzy drag her back to the dance studio. The dance teacher invited them all to audition for a musical and told Desiré, "I've got a part in mind for you". Desiré was ecstatic to be chosen. From then on, practising routines helped her lose a few pounds, but the dance teacher warned her not to shed too many because the part needed her "presence" as she called it. The teacher reminded her that no one has the perfect image that adverts project. The show went well and Desiré's success made her feel proud of herself.

Activities

- Create a collage of fashionable clothes.

- Using Worksheet 11, decide whether a girl and a boy your age might be shy, confident, happy or sad, hard or flexible, sharp or soft, etc.

- Talk about the messages put across by the way we dress.

- Write a rap on how girls feel about their image.

- Create a dance routine and/or rap and practise it.

Materials

Worksheet 11, teen fashion images, scissors, A3 card, felt tips, music player.

Discussion

- At the start of the story, Desiré was very critical of her body. Do most girls feel like this? Do you blame advertising? Or other influences?

- Desiré was scared she'd be mocked if she went to dance classes. What would encourage you to try dance, gym, sport or horse riding?

- Why do you think the skinny girl was rude to Desiré? At first, Desiré believed the unkind things. Has that happened to you? Would you stick up for a friend who was being attacked by nasty comments?

- What would you like to say to people, who advertise sexy clothes for young children? What do you think of pink for girls and blue for boys? Should parents set limits on young people's choice of clothes?

Reflections

- Desiré's critical views of her appearance are typical of lots of girls. Being saturated with media images of slim, toned, bodies, makes it hard to reach the perfection sold by advertising and media pressure.

- Having a friend to go with is probably the most encouraging way to try a new activity since if you both enjoy it, it will help you continue it.

- The skinny girl's rudeness was probably prompted by jealousy. It is easy to believe unkind remarks that cause some young people to get so self-conscious and anxious about imperfections, they stop eating.

- If someone makes a nasty comment to your friend, stick up for her by saying it's not true and that the nastiness belongs to the person it came from. Later think of more things to say to protect yourself from bullies.

- To advertisers selling sexy clothes for young children, one response could be, "Let her be a child, not a sex object!" Children need clothes they can run around in, comfortably, rather than just pose in.

- If toys are marketed to just one gender, it discourages the opposite one from playing with them. It creates the assumption that the toy is not for them so the child risks getting teased for playing with the wrong things. Boys caught playing with dolls fear mockery. Girls who like boys' stuff – trains and chemistry kits – risk getting called nasty names.

- When parents pay attention to what their children are wearing to social events they can encourage their teenage daughter to enhance one part of her body rather than every part at the same time (which risks getting nasty remarks or the kind of attention she doesn't want).

Pornography

Parents and caregivers worry when their pre-teen children take risks and disregard consequences. Young people don't want to disappoint the people responsible for them but they do want to know as much as possible in order to meet peer approval as well as adults' expectations. The Internet provides easy access however as McDonald-Brown et al. (2017) note, the rapid rise in social networking is making it harder for boys in the pre-teen age-group to keep up. Parents and teachers have an important role in helping them to develop self-efficacy that mitigates the risk of harm. Dines (2011) discovers that boys look at porn to find out the things they don't feel able to enquire of adults, such as how to go about sex and relationships. Story 35 illustrates that mistakes help us to learn from experience. Dimitri is caught downloading pornographic images and is devastated by his parents' reaction. Talking over what happened helps him to see the dangers and take up healthier pursuits.

How to use the story

- Read "Disaster for Dimitri" to explore young people's feelings about the pressures of meeting expectations from parents and teachers.

- To redress the child's dread of making mistakes, draw from examples of scientists, who view errors as vital to finding the formula that "works".

- Discuss the safe and unsafe use of Internet search engines.

- Invite anxious children, who are reluctant to talk about their worries, to write down particular anxieties and place their worries about the future into an envelope, which they can put aside for the time being.

Story 35: Disaster for Dimitri

The exams were looming but 14-year-old Dimitri was bored of studying. He disliked reading and hated writing essays. His birth Dad named him after a Greek god and now he was adopted his new Dad was nuts about history and wanted Dimitri to be a historian like him. His adoptive Mum hoped Dimitri would train to be a doctor, like her. Dimitri knew he stood no chance of either career but was scared of disappointing them in case they sent him packing. To tell the truth, he'd far rather play football except he wasn't good enough at that either. The competition to enter the local team was really strong! Lately, he'd skipped the most boring lessons, so was dreading his end of term report. He knew he'd get a hard time when his parents found out he'd been bunking off.

Dimitri snapped down the lid of his laptop then opened it again to check out a site he knew was supposed to be off limits. He'd just found one that looked interesting

when he heard a familiar tread on the stairs. Quietly cursing, he quickly shut the lid. Dad asked "What are you up to?" and passed him a flyer about a competition. The top prize was a weekend on an archaeology dig. Dad said, "I'll help you do the essay for it, don't worry!" This idea didn't remotely appeal to Dimitri but Dad had that gleam in his eye that said he'd already decided they'd win. It gave Dimitri a headache – it was so hard to say "no" to Dad. Willing him to go, Dimitri said "I'm trying to finish my homework."

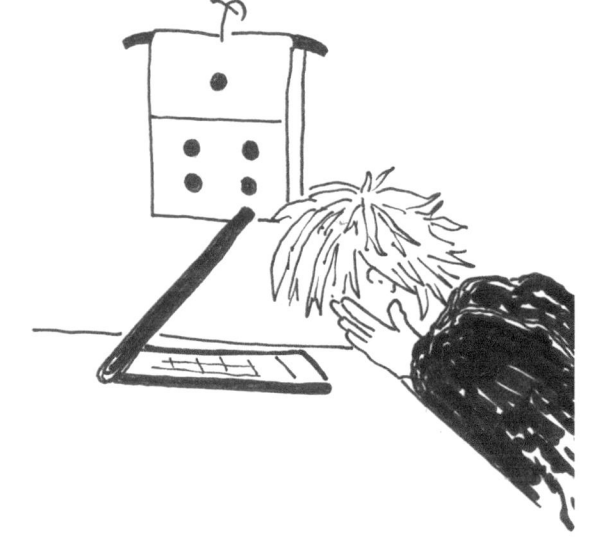

Finally Dad went and Dimitri returned to the screen he'd opened earlier. On impulse, he sent the link to his mate, Dante. That evening Dante's Dad came round to tell Dimitri's parents he'd seen shocking images on his son's computer and found 'dirty magazines' in his room. In the pile they'd found sketches drawn and signed by Dimitri. Overhearing, Dimitri felt his stomach cave in. His parents made grovelling apologies to Dante's Dad. As soon as he left, they went ballistic.

Dad shouted but Dimitri was surprised at how upset his Mum was. Their reactions seemed so extreme. Not sure what to say, Dimitri stayed silent to avoid further trouble. His parents got even madder, shouting things like, "You're such a disappointment to us! You're behaving like an animal!" Dimitri was devastated. He'd only looked at the forbidden sites out of curiosity, since Dante had told him everyone else did. That night, Dimitri couldn't sleep for thinking about what had happened and feeling terrified he'd get chucked out. Thinking he'd better make the decision for them, he got up, packed a rucksack and left the house. Dimitri started running but didn't know where to go. Around 5 a.m., he was frozen so he crept home and fell asleep, exhausted. At 8 a.m., Mum told him to get up for school. Wearily, he put his school uniform on but on the way, changed his mind and went to his auntie's house instead.

Ma Domino took one look at Dimitri and sent him to bed. She phoned the school to let them know he wasn't well enough to go in today, but decided to contact her sister later as she wouldn't miss him yet and Ma wanted to talk to him first. At 2 p.m. Dimitri woke up and went downstairs. He told her the whole story and how bad he was feeling. She listened not interrupting except to check she'd heard correctly. Eventually, Ma Domino asked him if he understood why porn sites were blocked. Dimitri said he reckoned it was because adults wanted to control young people. She replied that she'd feel very uncomfortable to see nude pictures of young girls she knew. Suddenly, Dimitri saw what she was meaning about porn, and he went bright red.

Ma Domino asked him how he was getting on at school. Dimitri said not very well but that he couldn't get Mum and Dad to accept he wasn't as clever as them. Ma said "Life's too short to spend doing things you hate!" She asked, "If you could choose what to do with your life, what would it be?" He shrugged. "Dunno – well I like drawing, and, yeah, animals." Ma suggested he go on an art course or phone the kennels to offer his help. She phoned his parents to invite them round and persuaded Dimitri to tell them which subjects he wanted to drop. When they arrived, Dimitri apologised for the trouble he'd caused and explained he hated not being as clever as them. Mum said she realised she ought to spend more time with him. Dad said he was disappointed that Dimitri had no enthusiasm for history, but agreed to let him do things he liked. Heaving a sigh of relief Ma Domino brought out some snacks!

Activities

- Act out a scene from each character's point of view.

- Share ideas for careers, based on your interests.

- Draw a poster advertising for part-time workers.

- Using Worksheet 12, attach pictures to each category and discuss the talents and personalities of each. What helps them succeed?

Materials

Worksheet 12, poster card, pencils, felt tip pens, spray paint, and crayons.

Discussion

- Dimitri didn't share his parents' ambitions – why do you think he couldn't tell them? Do your parents have ambitions for you?

- How do you think being adopted was affecting Dimitri?

- Dimitri wished he could be good at football. What sport, art or special interests would you love to be skilled at?

- Dimitri skipped lessons. Was he bored? Or scared he wasn't clever enough? Is that a problem for lots of young people? What helps you?

- What kind of Internet site do you think Dimitri was browsing? What risk did he take by sending the link to his mate?

- What effects does porn have on children and young people? When Dimitri ran away, he didn't think about what he might need. What should he have planned for? How did Ma Domino help him?

Reflections

- Dimitri was adopted. He was scared he would never meet his adoptive parents' ambitions for his future career. He dreaded disappointing them as he felt he'd never measure up even to competing in sport.

- However kind your adoptive parents are, if birth parents have let you go, it can leave you feeling "different" or less than desirable compared to children living with (natural) parents. Dimitri skipped lessons when he felt bored or didn't understand the lesson. He also felt there was so much that he didn't know about girls and stuff but really needed to.

- At age 10–14 there can be lots of risks from the Internet and social media chat rooms. Adults have been known to pose as teenagers to entice young people into conversation, then to meet them. Parents and caregivers worry about all these risks.

- Some boys like Dimitri look at porn sites to get information about how sex and relationships work because it's too hard to find someone to explain it to them. Sending the link led to Dimitri getting caught out.

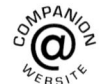

- There are magazines aimed at boys and young men that show pictures of girls in sexy poses. This implies that girls can be treated as property and have no rights to privacy, safety or ambitions for careers, interests and activities, which don't include men. They convey that men have an expectation of being in charge of women and girls.

- After Dimitri's parents got angry with him, he ran away, but forgot to take a waterproof and money, or to plan where to go. Ma Domino helped by giving him time to talk about all his worries. She encouraged him to think about what he liked doing, hoped to do, and also helped him to realise the dangers of porn and got him and his parents to talk openly.

7 Practice guidelines and case examples

Practice guidelines

This chapter provides guidelines and case examples to illustrate how this storytelling approach may be used by social workers, adoptive, foster and kinship parents, teachers and assistants, as well as by trained therapists.

Venue: Children, who have suffered repeated trauma, frequently operate at an emotionally younger age, especially when stressed. They will be hyper-vigilant to anticipated threat (see "Trauma" in Chapter 2). It is therefore very important that therapeutic intervention with fostered and adopted children is carried out in a safe place – usually the home where they are living. I find that it often helps to involve their caregiving parents. However some older children will prefer the privacy of school, which may be their safest place.

Choosing a story: Most of the stories in this book can easily be adapted to the opposite gender if you think this will make it easier for the child to relate to, however it is not essential. In work with a girl, for example, reading a story about a boy lends additional distance and privacy for the girl to say whether or not she identifies with the experiences described.

Avoid shaming: For a child, shame is debilitating and embarrassing. To avoid this risk, always try to relate to the child's feeling rather than to their "problem" behaviour (which shames them). Consider what motivates the child's particular inclinations, actions and reactions and view this as evidence of their courageous survival of adversity. For example the bossy child will have learned to assert him or herself in order to be heard, fed, comforted and sheltered. Use phrases such as "That must have been very hard for you!" and "I'm so impressed by how you did that!" "That's so clever!"

Build self-esteem: Writing down and making copies of the stories that children create will hugely reinforce their self-esteem and learning. The adult can type up the stories and add clip art illustrations or photos of the child's artwork, or the child can add their own pictures. The stories can be added to a folder for the child to keep, reread and reflect back on.

Allow the child to lead the activity. Imaginative play can have dreamlike qualities – the child explores the unconscious of possibilities. Non-cooperation is an indicator that the child has not had his/her pain heard and understood.

Be flexible: Children love to be naughty! Most of the time they are constrained by rules and conventions, but in play, the fictional context gives them permission to explore how to breach convention, e.g. outwit the adults,

Avoid asking lots of questions: We can't see inside a child's head so we don't actually know what they are thinking unless we ask. However for the child it can feel too intrusive to be questioned about their thoughts, feelings and actions (rather than a story character's). They may not know the answer anyway and it can spoil their trust in the adult. It is best to be led by the child.

Avoid telling children what you think they feel: You may well be wrong if you do so, and you may never find out how the child feels. Instead, try saying. "I wonder how this is making you feel?" Don't insist on an answer. The child will tell you directly or through play, if she or he trusts you (Sunderland, 2015).

Identity: Sometimes in imaginative play children explore the possibility of a duplicated version of themselves, such as a twin or someone looking like them and cases of mistaken identity. The child might also be preoccupied about the good/bad self, and be exploring the idea of "What if there is another me out there? Would that person be good or bad, desirable, or despicable?"

When children worry about looking different to their parents/caregivers: Some children are anxious about judgements they think are being made about them. Use open-ended questions to find out how the child views their family. There are all types of family and many siblings look different from each other. Caring parents turn up on time to collect children, have fun times holidays, trips etc.

Be patient: A child may defend against his feelings by appearing omnipotent and unaffected by the impact he has on others. If we validate his feelings, he will know his grievance is understood and will be more open to change.

Acknowledge a child's pain. Avoid platitudes and advice like "Get over it!"

Case examples

Example A: How a therapist can use the stories: Sophie, aged 13

Case history

In her birth family Sophie, White English, was dressed in dirty clothes, ate from the floor, slept in a dirty bed and suffered severe, persistent head lice. Her mother was abused in childhood, had learning difficulties, and suffered depression. As she rarely got up before noon, Sophie was left in her father's care. These parents were heavy drinkers. The police were often called to deal with the father's violence. After one fight, Sophie's mother locked father out and told the police he was sexually abusing Sophie. The mother admitted she had known about this abuse for two years, which the father had been replicating from his own childhood. Sophie was taken to foster care at age 7. She disclosed abuse but her father was never prosecuted due to lack of forensic evidence. Sophie lived for two years with a single carer and her three children then at age 9, was placed long term. Contact with her mother continued six times a year but reminded Sophie of past abuse and prompted her to seek closeness with other children in inappropriate ways.

Presenting issues

Sophie liked to be helpful and make her foster carers laugh. However neglect combined with genetic inheritance left her struggling to express herself, verbally. Therapy took place over a period of nearly three years because her teachers and caregivers found her especially difficult to deal with. She stole, showed reluctance to cooperate and jeered at the adults. Sophie was observed to disregard or fail to anticipate the consequences of her non-compliance. Her challenging behaviour was causing intense irritation, her fear and rage being displaced on to others. Its source needed to be understood. The aim of therapy was to enable Sophie to make sense of why she was in foster care. As the carer's agency was against intervention in the home, it took place in school. At the first session, Sophie was tearful following a troubling incident in the school cloakroom. She had picked up a drink and packet of crisps she'd found, and had drunk the cola but meant to return the crisps until one of her friends took the packet from her. This girl ate some crisps and passed the packet back to Sophie, who decided to eat a few then put the rest back. Sophie said the friend who "dobbed her in" had not owned up to her own part in this. Feeling friendless, Sophie was reluctant to face school the next day. The therapist acknowledged this dread and reassured her that everyone makes mistakes and as she didn't usually steal from her friends and was so upset, this showed that she knew right from wrong, therefore could be trustworthy. The therapist also reminded Sophie of all the friends she had made and the good report she'd been given the previous week.

Using the stories

The initial focus of intervention was on Sophie's life history. The therapist told Sophie she was loveable and helped her to understand the reason why her birth parents had been unable to look after her properly. This was because no one had loved or cared for them as children. Sophie engaged with immense enthusiasm in re-enacting scenes from her past. The therapist then moved on to stories about the Domino characters. Their fictional distance enabled Sophie to gain confidence to address the issues troubling her.

Story 23 – Daisy learns diplomacy

The first story was about a child's reluctance to back down from conflict. Sophie identified with this predicament. To increase her confidence in coping with a variety of problems, the therapist brought some problem pages from magazines for early teens. They dramatised some of these situations to give Sophie practice at ways to deal with problems and give advice:

Issue: Parents fighting
I'm 14 and my parents argue and shout all the time. Dad keeps swearing at Mum. I hear her crying herself to sleep every night. I've no one close enough to talk to about it. I've had huge rows with my parents and get so worked up I have asthma attacks. Dad tells me to stop looking for attention. I told Mum I felt like killing myself. She went mad and had to cancel her plans for the day to not leave me on my own. She loves me but Dad doesn't. I hate him. I don't want to live because I'm so unhappy. I'm crying as I write this. I feel so sick I've hardly eaten for two weeks. Please help!

Sophie advised: Ring Childline or find a teacher who will listen. They will advise you but try writing to your parents about how unhappy you are.

Issue: My friend steals my boyfriends:
My friend and I are 12. The problem is that every time I get a boyfriend she steals him off me. She's really pretty and all the boys are after her. I had quite a steady relationship with one boy and when she found out, she took him. It really upset

me. It's now happened four times with different boys. I don't want to keep her as a mate but I don't know how to tell her how I feel.

Sophie advised: Get someone to help you tell the girl how you feel. Then look for new friends who you can trust to not let you down.

Issue: Self-harm

I'm a huge fan of the actor, Jack Ryder. I think he's gorgeous and I know other girls do too but I've begun to do crazy things. Once I was watching the show and kept waiting and praying for Jack to appear on the screen so when he didn't I got very upset. I went to the kitchen, got a knife, carved a big heart into my arms and cut JR into the skin below the heart. It hurt me so much but it took away the hurt of not seeing him. Every night I cry for hours because I'm not with him. Please help me – I can't go on like this.

Sophie advised: You have to admit this is a fantasy. Talk to an adult you can trust who will listen and help or if you can't find one, ring Childline.

As teachers were continuing to complain that Sophie was poor at reading social situations, the therapist looked for a story to help Sophie with this.

Story 8 – Dotty tries to dominate

This story illustrates how a young person, craving her peers' acceptance and approval, finds herself trapped in awkward predicaments. The most traumatised children are likely to perceive their world as a dangerous and bewildering place and respond accordingly. On hearing the story, Sophie admitted to how hard she found it to guess at how people think or what could happen next. Having brought in a jewellery kit, the therapist invited Sophie to choose beads that represented feelings or ones that she just liked. While she was making a bracelet Sophie talked about complexities of navigating friendships. Encouraged to think ahead and please her family she began to plan a menu and write invitations for a meal. For a few weeks there were no complaints. Then Sophie was caught stealing sweets from her local shop. The therapist remarked that she must have wanted them badly and asked what led up to this. Sophie said her mates had bought sweets but she'd had no money left. The therapist sought a story to illustrate difficulties in resisting temptation.

Story 32 – Dan's dare

In this story a boy who steals a phone, learns how to be trustworthy. It illustrates the predicament known as FOMO – the fear of missing out – which affects many young people who crave to keep up with their more fortunate peers. Explaining the reason helps reduce the overwhelming pain of shame, and the story demonstrates that recovery from this is possible. After hearing it Sophie chose to play Bingo, a game of chance. She planned prizes, which players could win legitimately. The instances of her thefts reduced but the next week she was in trouble for avoiding a detention. Yet Sophie and her friend cornered the third culprit to explain why what they had been doing was wrong. This showed a development in her social conscience. Sophie told the therapist that she was often told off at school and anticipated this would carry on and stymie her ambition to work with a vet. The therapist drew an image of Sophie on a mountain between childhood and adulthood, and reassured her she would change. The next story chosen was on the power of peer pressure.

Story 30 – Decision for Dana

This story begins with the effects of cyber-bullying then describes a gang carrying out an act of racist vandalism. After reading the story, the therapist proposed a board game she'd made and named Celebrity Square. A dice is thrown and counters are moved that number of squares round the board of 100 squares. When a counter lands on a "Celebrity Square" the player picks up a card and answers questions on celebrities and their life styles. In the ensuing discussion Sophie said that she knew racism was wrong and described how she would resist being drawn into such a gang. Sophie felt that pop idols had social and moral responsibilities as role models, considering it was wrong for rich people to buy their way out of prison sentences. She began to follow news stories and design her own questions for the game.

Sophie wrote a letter to her idol, Justin Bieber: "Dear Justin, I am writing to ask for advice about the future and my new school. What should I do when I'm getting bullied and teased? Should I tell the teacher or keep it to myself? What if I'm getting told off? I normally laugh. Can you think of things I can say that won't get me into trouble? How can I have fun in lessons without getting told off and choose friends, who aren't a problem?" The therapist and Sophie devised lots of "What If" scenarios, to help Sophie think before acting.

Outcome

The therapist's calm manner soothed Sophie and enabled her to feel calmer in herself. Neuroscience reveals a warm, calm, accepting manner to be just as effective as physically holding in the way we do when we cuddle. A calm manner is especially important for traumatised children, who flinch at physical touch. The story-making approach enabled Sophie to make effective use of therapy and a successful transition to her new school. Sophie was able to sustain friendships having become far more self-aware. Her confidence in her abilities to survive socially and achieve ambitions is demonstrated in a poem that she compiled from choosing pertinent lines in her favourite songs:

Making my mind up

If you looked inside my brain
You'd find lots of things driving me insane.
I've been going round in circles, dizzy's all it made me
Never learn from my mistakes, that's what people tell me

You think I'm insecure
But I dunno what for
I'm turning heads when I walk through the door
Coz being the way I am is quite enough.

All the roads I had to walk
All the lights that flashed and led me to where I am
All I know is now I feel better than I did before
I make my mind up – don't mess with me any more.

Example B: How a social worker can use the stories: Finn, aged 11

Case history

Finn and his sister (who were White Irish) were taken to foster care due to neglect and domestic violence fuelled by their mother's and stepfather's addiction to alcohol and drugs, (their birth father had died some five years previously). They were returned to the mother but two years later went back to foster care. Finn and his sister had three more changes of placement prior to their current one, where they had lived for about a year and where the children were more supported.

Presenting issues

In his birth family Finn had taken a paternal role. Having looked after his alcoholic mother and younger sister, who had learning difficulties, he seemed much older than his age. Sibling rivalry was especially problematic. Finn showed coercive behaviour and was physically and emotionally abusive towards his sister – for instance he insisted on her getting changed if he thought her skirt was too short. Accustomed to parental violence Finn also tried to exert control over other children at school. Indeed until the current foster placement, he had never had a positive male role model to draw from. Finn wanted to return home to look after his birth Mum. His social worker, Carrie, hoped that ten (hour-length) sessions of life-story work at home would help Finn be reconciled to living long term with his current foster parents.

Using the stories

Finn was reserved, "buttoned up". Carrie searched for a story that Finn might relate to and would encourage him to talk about his feelings. Knowing he felt strongly protective of his sister, she aimed to address their relationship as a means of working towards giving him an explanation of his life story and the reasons why he was remaining long term in his foster placement. The first story focuses on the impact of loss experienced by a child whose brother disappears, causing her to realise how important he is to her.

Story 4 – Dorrie loses Davy

A key message of this story is that children are entitled to be treated equally. It invites them to reflect on their siblings' qualities and what they would miss if separated. After hearing the story, Finn painted a picture of an ocean then told a story about the arrival of a new fish and its encounter with a shark that dominates the ocean. The other fish are amazed at the new fish daring to challenge the shark's authority and expressing shocked disgust at the shark's rudeness before swimming away. Finn spoke of his wish to protect his sister from "sharks". This gave Carrie an opportunity to ask Finn if he was willing to hear more about the "sharks" he'd met and dealt with in the past.

As Finn appeared cautiously willing to hear more about his family, Carrie produced a life map she'd drawn of the houses he'd lived in. They worked out the order in which Fin had been to each house. Aware that Finn had moved between his parents and grandparents for a while, for the next session, Carrie chose the story of a girl, who becomes fed up with being in two families:

Story 1 – Dora's dilemma

This story invites discussion on the responsibilities of children and adults and the efforts that older children often make to look after their younger siblings when the adults aren't around. Dora is helped to think of ways to be reconciled to her family being split up. On hearing this story, Finn recalled times of having to protect his sister from assaults by Mum's partner. Carrie empathised and explained why it was so important for him and his sister to be safe, able to grow up without living in perpetual fear. She invited him to draw a picture of his family home. When Finn finished she suggested he turn it over and divide it into jigsaw pieces that could be cut out. Instead Finn chose to tell a story about the family home being crashed into by a drunk driver. As his birth Mum had a car accident when drunk, Carrie remarked how frightening this must have been for him as well as Mum – it showed just how unwell she had been.

The next story Carrie chose was on the stress of coping with mental illness.

Story 13 – Dodgems

This story is about two children placed in care after having looked after their mentally ill mother and endured her relentless criticism. Her fragility meant they had missed school and social opportunities. Typically, the children blame themselves for what they assume to be their fault. On hearing the story "Dodgems" Finn remarked that it was very like his life story. Carrie reflected that now Finn was having a very different time and enjoying better care, he would grow up able to make better choices than those his parents made. In reference to the discussion points, as he reflected on the ups and downs of life Finn drew a fairground scene complete with rides. He admitted how impossible he found it to risk showing any weakness. Finn then turned the fairground into a theme park, where a show takes place. The show featured a brave knight, who queried the guard's right to boss him around. The knight is repeatedly threatened by an evil goblin. Carrie asked the "knight" how this felt. In the role of the "knight" (Finn) told her he was forced to use his wits in the battle for survival. Carrie recognised the constant threats as representing Finn's compulsive hyper vigilance. In fictional contexts, the role of "hero" gives the opportunity to try out heroic qualities of stoicism and desire to help others.

Outcome

Finn gained a positive understanding of his life story. He enjoyed hearing stories and creating his own. The stories being fictional enabled him to explore his feelings without fear of embarrassing exposure. His own stories demonstrated his wish to strive forward and try his hardest. Seeing them typed up and illustrated enhanced his self-esteem. Finn began to show improved control of his affect (expression of feeling). In evaluation, he wrote that he understood why he and his sister had not been safe in their birth family. Finn was now showing more affection to his foster parents and had ceased blaming himself for the unfortunate circumstances of his time in birth family. The story-based therapy helped him to realise that everyone makes mistakes and once the mistakes have happened they can be learned from.

Example C: How an adoptive parent can use the stories: Kayla, aged 11

Case history

Kayla was of dual heritage – her father, Black Caribbean and her mother White British. Kayla was highly traumatised by neglect and physical abuse by Mum's partners during extensive domestic violence. Her birth parents had disruptive, difficult childhoods. Her father was alcohol dependent and her mother had a series of abusive relationships and relied on drugs and alcohol to get by. At 3 years of age, Kayla was admitted to hospital with severe injuries, and in abject terror. She was 4 years old when a police raid of the home found Kayla watching a pornographic DVD while her mother was taking drugs. A year later a further assault by a former partner led to Kayla and her brother being taken to (White British) foster carers, who later adopted them.

Presenting issues

The effects of the traumas suffered by Kayla abated for a time but resurfaced when she began to experience unkind taunts in school. Believing these taunts, Kayla became extremely distressed. Hating herself, she cut her wrists, wrote suicide messages and refused to go out, too scared to leave her place of safety. Adoptive Dad, Len, became highly stressed with the ensuing conflict. Adoptive Mum, Louise, sought professional help without success so looked for books to help Kayla as best she could. Louise designated an hour a week at the dining table to share stories and encourage Kayla to engage in various creative activities to help reduce her stress.

Using the stories

Louise knew that stories illustrated ways to manage life's challenges. Aware that Kayla was behind at school she sought one that would address her feelings about this. Louise found a story about a boy, who feels worthless, until on making a friend he is helped to gain a sense of pride in himself.

Story 7 – Dudley who thought he was Dud

This story illustrates the distressing impact of verbal abuse (see Chapter 1) and how helping someone brings the child friendship and acceptance. Kayla recognised that Dudley's feelings and experiences matched her own. She and Louise enacted a scene in which Dudley is told off for not completing a task. Empathising with the distress this causes, Louise encouraged Kayla to tell her what she found hardest at school. Kayla felt that the worst part was being unable to tell the time. As Kayla struggled to distinguish sections of hours, Louise drew a big circle and invited her to illustrate activities related to each hour. Kayla worked out that certain TV theme tunes were a useful guide to knowing what time it was and sought other clues to telling the time. Even so Kayla continued to dread school. Complaining of being bullied, she interpreted others' advice and the way they looked at her, as putdowns. Louise knew these girls and was fairly confident that they were trying to help Kayla. Recognising that lack of confidence and fear of ridicule were impeding Kayla and causing her to worry perpetually, Louise searched for a story to illustrate different ways to interpret and understand others' motivations.

Story 34 – Dancing for Desiré

In this story a girl, who believes she's too fat to attend a dance class is persuaded to go to one, Mockery from a rival classmate upsets her until praise from the teacher enables her to enjoy dancing. On hearing the story, Kayla absorbed the message that having her talent recognised helped the girl to enjoy it. Though not keen to attend dance classes, Kayla asked for a bigger sketchbook and drew pictures from her favourite films. With encouragement, a story of empowerment emerged from her drawing of a mythical creature. Kayla's story illustrated that the motivation for denigration was to take power but she took out her frustrations on Len. Kayla asserted that only her real Dad (birth father, who was deceased) would understand her. To help Kayla realise that in being so hard on Len, she was blaming him for the men, who had let her down in the past, Louise read her a story about divided loyalties.

Story 2 – Dylan's dread (divided loyalties)

This story focuses on the anxieties of a young person weighed down by responsibilities he took on for his struggling family. As Louise and Kayla enacted scenes from it, Kayla realised that she knew Len could be trusted not to betray Louise in the way Dylan was scared his Dad might. Louise asked Kayla if she wanted things with Len to carry on getting worse or better. Kayla admitted that she wished things were better and at Louise's suggestion, wrote a letter to Len, listing things she liked and appreciated about him. Len was touched. Sensing that Kayla needed to make sense of how she came to be adopted, Louise was nonetheless, wary of being judged as too blaming of birth parents. She looked for a story to sensitively illustrate Kayla's predicament, without being too close a replica of her life story.

Story 3 – Darma's despair

This story illustrates the traumatic impact of abuse and violence on the young person's learning capacity and relationships. Things get worse until her caregiver acquires the facts of her history and realises its impact on Darma. On hearing the story, Kayla recognised the character's experiences and felt relieved to have an explanation as to why she struggled with relationships and learning. Louise obtained detailed information on Kayla's life story and wrote a simplified version of it. After hearing her adoptive Mum's version, Kayla celebrated adoption by creating a collage of her life, friends and interests.

Outcome

Relationships between Kayla and Len improved. Kayla's self-harming ceased. The time spent on this work enhanced her confidence in her parents' emotional availability. Still, it is a long and slow process to heal from trauma. Kayla needed professional help to adjust her propensity to blame her birth Mum, whilst idolising her birth Dad, who had been just as culpable.

Example D: How a teacher/mentor can use the stories: Greg, aged 10

Case history

Greg's mother is White English and father Jamaican/Indian. At 6 years of age he was taken from his birth mother due to neglect, alcohol abuse, and domestic violence involving his father and mother's subsequent partners. Greg was placed in foster care with his older disturbed sister, who blamed him for their removal from home and abused him physically and emotionally. She moved to a residential home but Greg then had three more foster placements. Unfortunately his caregivers had little time for him. Greg blamed himself for everything that went wrong and worried constantly about his birth mother (who extended family and social workers were unable to contact).

Presenting issues

Greg showed compliance in a desire to appease, but frustrated his caregivers by refusing to make choices, to avoid causing offence. Following the loss of important relationships Greg was finding it difficult to trust any adults. His past trauma left him hyper-vigilant and unable to keep still. His sleep was regularly disturbed by intrusive memories. Greg also suffered high anxiety in groups.

Using the stories

Terri, an experienced teacher of children with special needs and Special Educational Needs Coordinator, had met Greg's birth Mum and knew his history. She arranged six sessions of creative play and story making to encourage Greg to express his feelings.

Story 20 – Drumming for Dibs

This story is about a boy, who had endured multiple foster placements and felt embarrassed about being frequently in trouble at school. Terri read the story and drew from the discussion points to invite Greg's view on Dibs having so many foster placements. Greg replied, *"It sucks!"* Encouraging him to tell her more, Terri invited Greg to create a musical instrument from the junk materials she'd found. He worked enthusiastically making a guitar until a disparaging remark from a passing teacher discouraged him. Greg immediately rubbished his efforts. Terri tried to reassure him that the guitar was actually very neat. She explained that the whole point of play is to let you experiment, mess about and find out what works so there is no need for perfection. Greg shrugged, irritable and disappointed. Acknowledging his feelings, Terri said, *"You really wanted to make this model and now its like nothing is working for you. I'm wondering if this is a feeling left from the many times you've been let down."* Knowing how difficult it is for children with low self-esteem to cope with imperfection that (in their perception) confirms their sense of inadequacy, Terri looked for a story that reflected some aspects of Greg's life story.

Story 22 – Dusty's Distress

In this story, the mother's alcohol dependency and lifestyle leads to her two daughters being taken to foster care in separate places. The younger sibling shows signs of alcohol addiction and gets angry with her older sister for having abandoned her. Greg identified with the feelings of the older one, who is blamed for events that were beyond her control or influence. Terri asked Greg if he'd like to write a letter to his Mum or his sister. He wrote one to each of them and asked to visit his sister. Terri emailed the social worker, who enabled this contact. Concerned that Greg was vulnerable to peer influence, Terri sought a story that would address the risks he was facing in school.

Story 31 – Dean escapes the "Nos"

This story describes a boy who is enrolled into a gang and gets caught by the police. After hearing the story, Greg didn't want to talk about it but used toy figures to enact a violent battle in which the King battles with an alien and a pirate sneaks up and slices off their ankles. The King had a gun, while the aliens had an entire army so the King's defences (like Greg's) soon crumble. The fast action made it difficult for Terri to know which character was on which side – good or evil. It reflected Greg's confusion as to whether anyone could be trusted and his struggle to decide on the outcome. Terri expressed empathy for dilemma of each of the main characters. She asked the King (Greg) what it was like for him to be in this battle. The "King" admitted he was scared and didn't know what to think. Terri then asked the King how he would like the story to end. Greg decided to have the aliens "turn good" and realise it is better to have friends and tell jokes, rather than be in conflict. This outcome suggested Greg's anxiety to please and win approval. Although Greg had expressed various aspects of the conflicts preoccupying him Terri was aware that he had said little directly about his traumatic past. She sensed that the right story might invite him to make connections with his own feelings.

Story 15 – Dixie's devastation

This story describes the debilitating experience of post-traumatic stress for a young asylum seeker, who arrives in a new place, alone, starving, homeless and unable to speak the language. Instinctively Greg went on to play out his own traumatic experience, creating the following story of a war:

> *The English army were relying on camouflage for protection. A captain is killed, so "crazy guys" are in charge. Soldiers play "dead" (to avoid getting killed). Missiles fly between rival armies. When all the soldiers sleep, an assassin shoots the opposition with tranquillisers. In the end the English win.*

Terri praised the courage and common sense of the soldiers. She remarked, *"They must be tired!"* Greg told her how scary his life with his parents had been – so much fighting and so many injures. He wished he could sleep better at night. Terri empathised and Greg felt relieved that she understood how much he struggled with everything. Later Terri spoke with his teacher about these fictional battles, which she recognised as a metaphor for the domestic violence Greg had witnessed. Terri guessed the killing of the "army captain" symbolised Greg's experience of police officers' inability to control his parents' violence, freeing the "crazy" ones to do their worst. The assassin's attack seemed to represent the child's fear of sleeping in case something frightening should happen. Terri remarked that Greg had used weapons for strength and protection rather than for killing. Concerned that Greg's contriving to have the English army win was another way of appeasing adults with an acceptable outcome, Terri sought a story exploring the fear of confrontation.

Story 24 – Donald's story

In this story about fears of racist bullying, confrontation from a bully afflicts the main character, Donald, until a new peer's friendly smile encourages him to make friends. Greg's mixed heritage made him vulnerable to unkind teasing about his thick curly hair. To invite him to explore his sense of identity, Terri introduced animal (hand) puppets. The play started with each character stating how they came to be named. Frog (Greg) then accused Rat of stealing his eggs. Rat (Terri, following Greg's directions) denied this. Greg then took up Chimp, who shows off and is rude to the others. When Squirrel (Terri) objects, Cheeky Dog (Greg) announces, "I'm special!" A fight erupted over who is king then who has the strongest teeth. Terri sensed that Greg was remembering fights with his sister, who had victimised him. In his latest foster placement he was experiencing conflict with a younger child. Terri said, "That girl has a mother she can rely on. Its so much harder for you!" The puppet play freed Greg to practise recognising the kind of non-verbal signals implicit in social communication, which he had missed learning as a young child.

For the final session, Terri lit candles to represent Greg and his family. Greg took the opportunity to say how he felt towards each member of his family. He said he loved them but wished they had kept him safe and were still there for him. After this, to provide nurture, Terri produced some biscuits to ice and decorate.

Outcome

Greg engaged in these sessions with huge enthusiasm. He showed courage in sharing frightening memories of his past life. Once inclined to idealise his mother, he gained a more balanced appreciation of her responsibility as a parent, who let him down. Greg hugely enjoyed nurture play he had missed in his chaotic family of origin. Desperate for a sense of belonging he was keen to win approval. This therapeutic play enables children such as Greg to enjoy an interested adult's undivided attention and to develop their imagination. Having their experiences validated enables the child to process feelings and move on to make more satisfying and reciprocal relationships in the future.

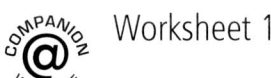

Organising my life

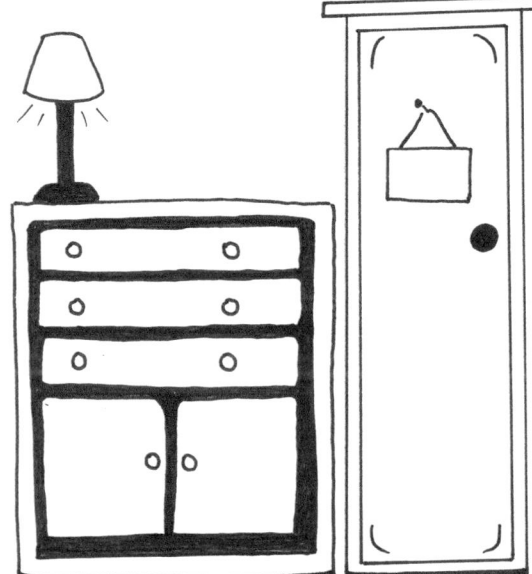

What I will keep in each drawer?

1..

2..

3..

How I will organise my clothes in my wardrobe or room?

....

....

....

Things to take in my school bag each day. Where will I keep it?

....

....

....

What time will I start and finish my homework?...

Which days will I see my friends after school?...

Which day is my special interest group/club?..

Worksheet 2

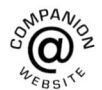

Things I could say to bullies

"Get lost!" or, "It takes one to know one!"

"I'm so glad I don't think like you do!"

"It's a shame all you can talk about is such a load of rubbish! Your mind must be a sewer!"

"You think you're so funny, you should just listen to yourself!"

"Luckily this doesn't worry me like it seems to bother you!"

"Well, time's moved on and so have I. Shame I can't say the same about you!"

Now add your own ideas:

....

....

....

....

....

....

....

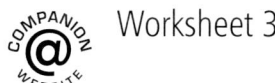

Memory jar

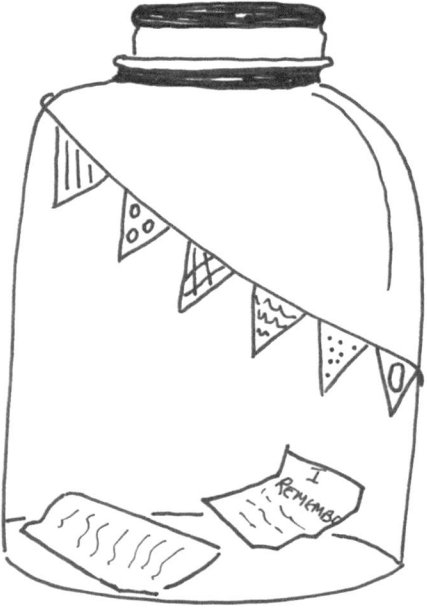

Draw or write things you'd like in your memory jar

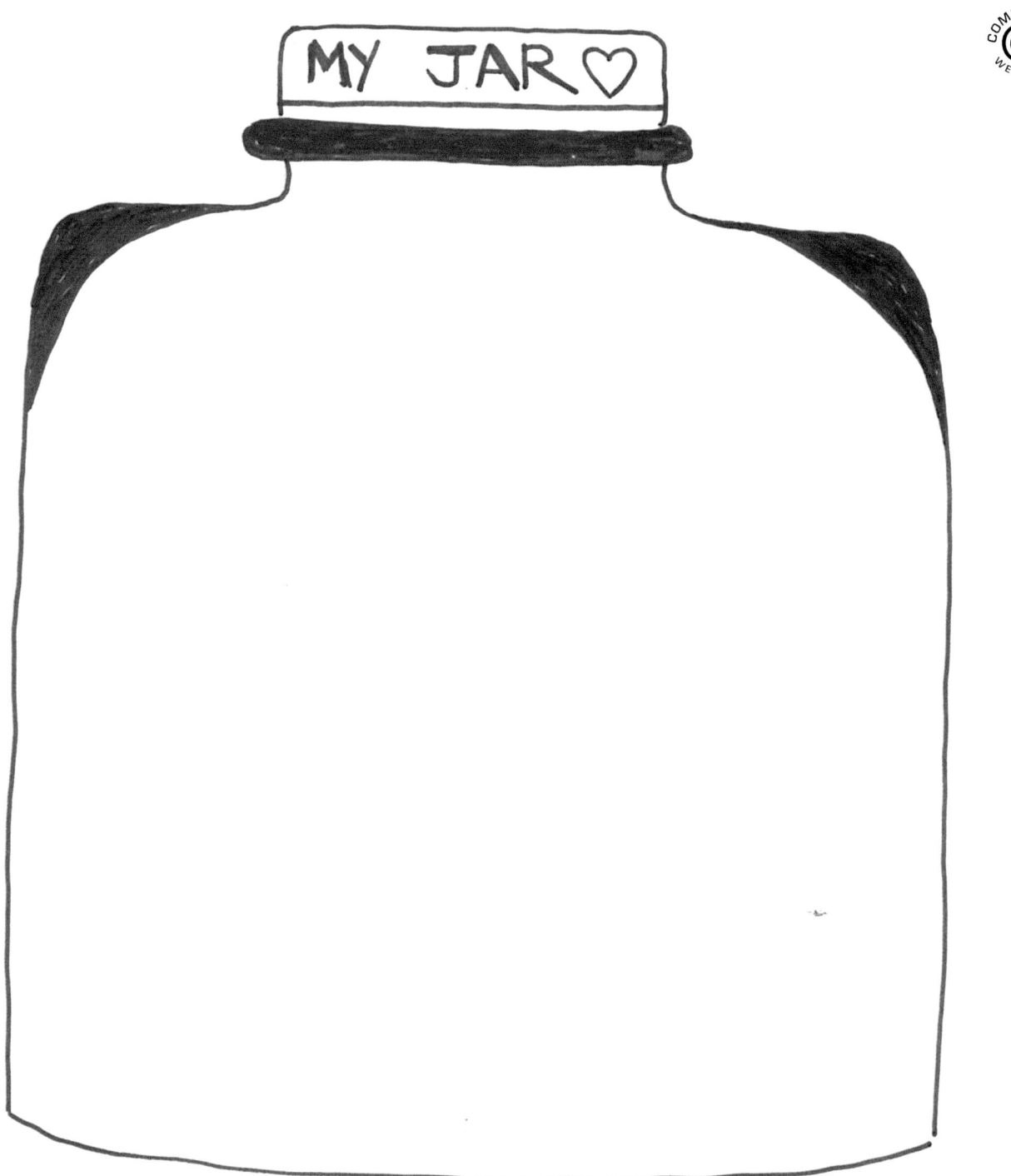

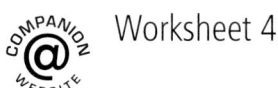

Map of your area

Draw a map of where you live. Add places that are likely to be of interest to recently arrived refugees. Include the advice centre, surgery, café, swimming pool, football pitch, park, library, theatre, cinema, school, and other important features, perhaps a particular shop. Illustrate the map with symbols such as a "book" to portray the library and a "first aid" cross on the medical centre.

My town/village is called...................

Worksheet 5

Date:......................................

Menu

Starter

Main Course

Dessert

Drinks

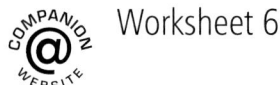

Invitation cards

You are invited to dinner

by

....

On this date

....

At this address

....

....

....

At this time

....

Please reply

Name:..

Worksheet 7

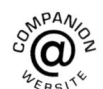

Problem page

1. Mate hate

I'm 11 and I've made friends with someone who everyone disses. I'm scared my other friends will be horrible to this person and I don't want to tell them that people bitch about them. I'm stuck. What can I do?

2. Feeling bullied

I'm 12 and am in a gang. We do everything together but I get picked on more than the others. They usually say they're only messing around but it hurts my feelings. How can I get them to back off?

3. No confidence

I'm 13 and I feel really self-conscious. I don't like anything about myself. What can I do to feel more confident?

4. Divisive friends

I was hanging out with a mate who'll be coming to my school but she's (he's) asking me to ditch my best friend there. What should I do?

5. Left out

I have fun with my friends but I think they keep a lot of things from me. When I ask what they're talking about they say it's none of my business. How can I find out what's going on and stop this happening?

6. Smothered

I really like my boyfriend but he won't let me spend time with my friends. I'm scared he'll dump me if I see them without him there.

7. Fallout

My best friend is suddenly barely talking to me. She's acting like she doesn't want to be with me, even when we're doing fun things. She says she's depressed and it's just a phase. How can I make her smile?

8. Photo sharing

A 16-year-old boy who I fancy has asked me to send him photos of myself, topless. I'm 13 but he thinks I'm older. If my parents knew they'd go ballistic, but I don't want to lose him.

9. Pestered for sex

I'm 13 and on the pill. I've told my boyfriend it's not for the reason he thinks but I'm worried he might take advantage. What should I do?

10. Scary stepdad

My friend's stepdad picks on her but treats his own children like royalty. She's really scared of him but her Mum sides with her stepdad so my friend has no one she can tell n her family. What can she do?

Answers

1. **Mate Hate**: You could ask your friends why they don't like this person you think is really cool. Say, "S/he's my friend and I'd like you to meet her/him" Its best to ask before turning up with the friend.

2. **Bullied:** They are probably doing this just to get a reaction. Try saying, "That's not even funny!" Don't take it personally or lower your standards by retaliating and making the situation escalate.

3. **No confidence**: This happens to a lot of young people. Focus on the things you are ok with; look after your skin and hair. Wear clothes you feel comfortable in and suit you. Don't try to be someone you're not. Show interest in others. Their problems can make yours seem smaller.

205

4. **Jealous friend:** Tell your friend that when s/he comes to your school you're very happy to be mates but it won't change the friendships you already have. Help your friend see that it would be unfair to drop your other friends and promise to introduce him/her to your schoolmates.

5. **Left out:** Let your friends know you feel awkward, embarrassed when they leave you out. Explain that you don't mean to be nosy. You just want to feel included as their friend. If they continue to not consider your feelings, you might want to find some new friends.

6. **Smothered:** Your feelings are just as important as your boyfriend's. Explain that you like to spend time with him but need time for yourself. If he puts you under pressure, you may be better off without him.

7. **Fallout:** You are trying to be there for her and it may be just a phase, but if your friend is depressed, s/he may need to go to a doctor or school nurse or guidance teacher, who'll find ways to help her.

8. **Photo-sharing:** You have to expect that pictures go viral quickly, which can be embarrassing and give you a kind of reputation you won't want. It is a good idea to tell a parent or teacher you trust, so they can warn the boy to back off, and if he persists, inform his parents.

9. **Pestered for sex:** The pill is designed to protect you from pregnancy but it can be prescribed for other reasons such as painful periods. Remind your boyfriend as many times as necessary, that you are not ready to have sex yet and that it is illegal under the age of 16.

10. **Scary stepdad**: Encourage your friend to talk to a relative and if this is not possible, to tell a teacher she trusts, or to phone Childline for advice. She has rights and should not be made to feel afraid in her own home. You are doing your best to support her by being concerned.

Worksheet 8

Write a poem about friendship and decorate it

Worksheet 9

Allotment shed

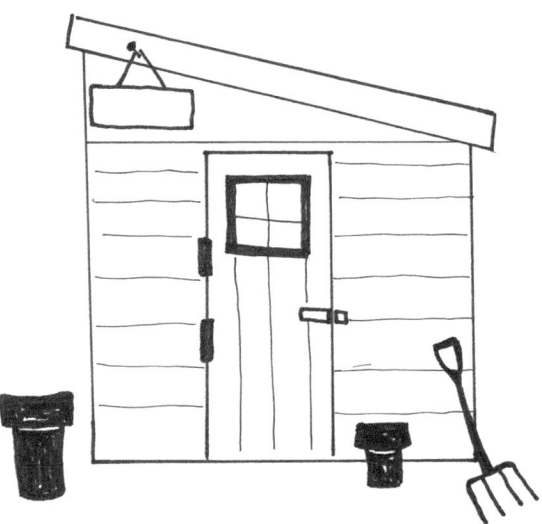

Use the space below to draw your own shed or den and some of the things that you would like to keep inside it.

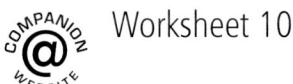

Compliments

In the bubbles write a compliment that a girl and boy can pay each other

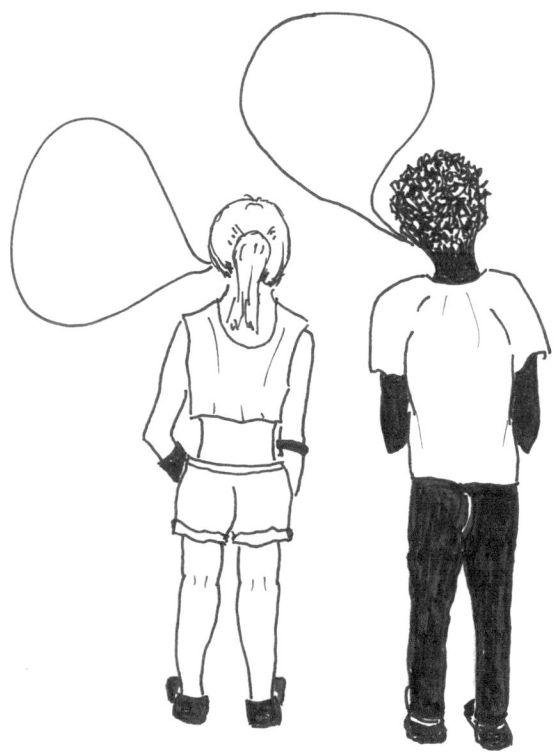

Worksheet 11

Young people – characteristics

Attach picture and list characteristics

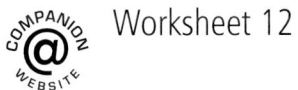

Famous people

Sports personality   Singer

TV presenter   Celebrity

Cartoon character/s

Bibliography

Ahern, N.R., Sauer, P. and Thacker, P. (2015) Risky behaviours and social networking sites: How is YouTube influencing our youth? *Journal of Psychosocial Nursing and Mental Health Services*, 53:10, 25–29.

Andel, P. (2019) *Thinking Seriously about Gangs: Towards a Critical Realist Approach.* Cham, Switzerland: Palgrave Macmillan.

Baldry, A.C. Sorrentino, A. and Farrington, D.P. (2018) Post-traumatic symptoms among Italian preadolescents involved in school and cyber bullying and victimization. *Journal of Child and Family Studies*, 28, 2358–2364.

Beckoff, M. (2007) *The Emotional Lives of Animals: A Leading Scientist Explores Animal Joy, Sorrow and Empathy – and why they Matter.* Novato, CA: New World Library.

Bhopal, K. (2018) *The Myth of a Post-Racial Society.* Bristol: Bristol University Policy Press.

Bindel, J. (2014) *An Unpunished Crime? The Lack of Prosecutions for FGM in the UK.* New Culture Forum. Available at: www.west-info.eu/uk-doesnt-punish-fgms-perpetrators/julie-bindel-an-unpunished-crime-the-lack-of-prosecutions-for-female-genital-mutilation-in-the-uk-2014/.

Blakemore, S. (2018) *Inventing Ourselves: The Secret Life of the Teenage Brain.* London: Doubleday.

Booker, C. (2004) *The Seven Basic Plots.* London: Blooomsbury.

Bowlby, J. (1989) *A Secure Base.* London: Tavistock.

Boyd, B. (2009) *On the Origin of Stories, Evolution, Cognition and Fiction, USA.* Cambridge, MA: Harvard University Press.

Boyd, B. (2018) The evolution of stories: From mimesis to language, from fact to fiction. *WIRE's Cognitive Science*, 9, 1–16.

Carey, T. (2016) *Girls Uninterrupted: Steps for Building Stronger Girls in a Challenging World.* London: Icon Books Ltd.

Caw, J. and Sebba, J. (2014) *The Team Parenting Approach for Children in Foster Care: a Model for Integrated Therapeutic Care.* London: Jessica Kingsley.

Childline (Independent 8.1.14).

Coholic, D. (2010) *Arts Activities for Children and Young People in Need: Helping children to Develop Spiritual Awareness and Self-Esteem.* London: Jessica Kingsley.

Bibliography

Coman, W., Dickson, S., McGill, L. and Rainey, M. (2016) Why am I in care? A model for communicating with children about entry to care that promotes psychological safety and adjustment. *Adoption and Fostering*, 40:1, 49–59.

De Heering, A. Rossian, B., and Maurer, D. (2012) Developmental changes in face recognition during childhood: Evidence from upright and inverted faces. *Cognitive Development*, 17:1, 17–27.

De Thierry, B. (2017) *The Simple Guide to Child Trauma*. London: Jessica Kingsley.

Degli-Esposti, M., Humphreys, D.K., Jenkins, B.M., Gasparrini, A., Poolley, S., Eisner, N. and Bowes, L. (2019) Long-term trends in child maltreatment in England and Wales, 1858–2016: an observational, time-series analysis. *The Lancet*, 4:3, 148–156.

DfE (2017) The National FGM Centre: an evaluation.

DfE (2018) Improved Mental Health support for children in care. Press release, 13 June 2018. Available at: www.gov.uk/government/news/improved-mental-health-support-for-children-in-care.

Dines, G. (2011) *Pornland: How Porn has Hijacked our Sexuality*. Boston, MA: Beacon Press.

Dixon, S., Shacklock, J. and Leach, J. (2019) Female genital mutilation: Barriers to accessing care. *The BMJ*, 364, 1921.

Ehmke, R. (2019) How using social media affects teenagers. *Child Mind Institute* 8:6. Available at: https://childming.org/article/howusing-social-media-affects-teenager/.

Fahlberg, V. (1994, 2008) *The Child's Journey Through Placement*. London: BAAF.

Festi, R. and Quandt, T (2017) Cyber Bullying. *Wiley Online Library*. Available at: https://doi.org/10.1002/9781118783764.wbieme0171.

Frydenburgh, E. (2008) *Adolescent Coping: Advances in Theory, Research and Practice* (2nd edn). London: Routledge/Taylor & Francis Group.

Fuentes, M.J., Bernedo, I.M., Salas, M.D. and Garcia-Martin, M.A. (2018) What do foster families and social workers think about children's contact with birth parents? A focus group analysis. *International Social Work*, 62:5, 1416–1430.

Gerhardt, S. (2004) *Why Love Matters: How Love Shapes the Baby's Brain*. Hove: Brunner-Routledge.

Gilbert, E. and Sinclair, P. (2019) *Devastating After Effects: Anti-Knife Crime Sessions*. Barkway: The Flavasum Trust.

Gray, L.A. (2020) Lifting the Veil: Why Children are Still Getting Married in America. *Independent,* 16.4.20.

Grotevant, H., Reuter, M. Von Korff, L., Gonzalez, C. (2011) Post-adoption contact, adoption communicative openness, and satisfaction with contact as predictors of externalizing behavior in adolescence and emerging adulthood. *Journal of Child Psychology and Psychiatry,* 52:5, 529–536.

Harari, Y.N. (2014) Sapiens; A Brief History of Humankind. London: Harvill Secker.

Heald, A., Vida, B., Farman, S. and Bhugra, D. (2018) The Leave vote and racial abuse towards Black and Ethnic communities across the UK: the impact on mental health. *Journal of the Royal Society of Medicine,* 111:5, 158–161.

Holmwood, C. (2021 in press) Making a dramatic story out of a crisis – a response to Covid 19. In Jennings, S., Holmwood, C. and Jackties, S. (eds) *The Routledge International Handbook of Storytelling and Therapeutic Stories.* London: Routledge.

House of Commons Science and Technology Committee (2019) Impact of social media and screen-use on young people's health, Fourteenth Report of Session (2017–2019) Report together with formal minutes relating to the report. HC822.

Hunnikin, L.M., Wells, A. E., Ash, D.P. and van Goozen, S.A.M. (2019) The nature and extent of emotion recognition and empathy impairments in children showing disruptive behavior referred into a crime prevention programme. *European Child and Adolescent Psychiatry.* Available at: https://link.springer.com/content/pdf/10.1007/s00787-019-01358-w.pdf.

Independent (22.8.13) Children are overweight and under exercising, NHS (2013).

Independent (21.1.20) The covert racism faced by minority ethnic teachers, reported by Eleanor Busby, Education correspondent.

Jay, A. (2013) Independent Inquiry into Child Sexual Exploitation in Rotheram, 1997–2013, commissioned by Rotherham Metropolitan Borough Council.

Jennings, S. (2012) The roots of ritual theatre: An anthropological perspective. In Schrader, C. (ed.) *Ritual Theatre: The Power of Dramatic Ritual.* London: Jessica Kingsley.

Jones, C. (2015) Sibling relationships in adoptive and foster families: A review of the international research literature. *Children and Society,* 30:4, 324–334.

Keen, D.V., Fonsecca, S. and Wintgens, A. (2008) Selective mutism: A consensus based care pathway of good practice. *Archives of Disease in Childhood,* 93:10, 838–844.

Bibliography

Kelly, L and Karsna, K. (2017, updated 2018), Measuring the scale and changing nature of child sexual abuse and child sexual exploitation, Centre of Expertise on Child Sexual Abuse, London Metropolitan University.

Kelly, M. and McBride, A.B. (2019) The forensic evaluation. In Carrion, Victor G. (ed.) *Assessing and Treating Youth Exposed to Traumatic Stress*. Washington, DC: American Psychiatric Publishing.

Kim, J.R. and Tucker, A. (2019) The inclusive family support model: Facilitating openness for post-adoptive families. *Child and Family Social Work*, 25:1, 173–181.

Kokkinos, C.M., Kakarini, S. and Kolovou, D. (2015) Relationships among shyness, social competence, peer relations and theory of mind among pre-adolescents. *Social Psychology of Education*, 19: 117–133.

Kopelman, L.M. (2016) The forced marriage of minors: A neglected form of child abuse. *Journal of Law, Medicine and Ethics*, 44:1, 173–181.

Kubler, Ross E. (1969) *On Death and Dying*. London: Routledge.

Lehrer, J. (2009) *How We Decide*. New York: Houghton Mifflin Harcourt.

Linares, T., Singer, L, Kirchner, H.L., Short, E.J., Min, M.O., Hussey, P. and Minns, S. (2005) Mental health outcomes for cocaine-exposed children at six years of age. *Journal of Pediatric Psychology*, 31:1, 85–97.

Lu, A. and Johnson, K. (2019) The UK and Ireland incidence of Foetal Alcohol Syndrome (FAS): a new study. *Advances in Dual Diagnosis*, 12:1/2, 99–102.

Luke, N., Sinclair, I., Woolgar, M and Sebba, J. (2014) *What Works in Preventing and Treating Poor Mental Health in Looked After Children?* Rees Centre Oxford: NSPCC.

McDonald-Brown, C., Laxman, K. Hope, J. (2017) Sources of support and mediation online for 9–12 year old children. *E Learning and Digital Media*, 14:1–2, 52–71.

Mackes, N.K., Golm, D., Sarkar, S., Kumsta, R., Rutter, M., Fairchild, G., Metha, M.A. and Sonuga-Barke, E.J.S. (2020) Early childhood deprivation is associated with alterations in adult bone structure despite subsequent environmental enrichment. *PNAS*, 117:1, 641–649.

Manning, C. and Gregoire, A. (2009) Effects of parental mental illness on children. *Psychiatry*, 8:1, 7–9.

Matthews, T., Holt, V., Sahin, S., Taylor, A. and Griksaitis, D. (2019) Gender dysphoria in looked after and adopted young people in a gender identity development service. *Clinical Child Psychology and Psychiatry*, 24:1, 112–128.

Mehrabian, A. (ed.) (2017) *Nonverbal Communication*. Abingdon: Routledge.

Moore, J. (2012*) Once Upon a Time: Stories and Drama to Use in Direct Work with Fostered and Adopted Children*. London: CoramBAAF.

Moore, J. (2014) Emotional Problem Solving Using Stories Drama and Play. Buckingham: Hinton House.

Moore, J. (2019) The storying spiral: A narrative-dramatic approach to life story therapy with adoptive/foster families and traumatised children. *International Journal of Play*, 8:2, 204–218.

Moore, J. (2020) *Narrative and Dramatic Approaches to Children's Life Story with Foster, Adoptive and Kinship Families: using the Theatre of Attachment Model*. London: Routledge.

Moore, J. Anderson-Warren, M. and Kirk, K. (2017) Dramatherapy and Psychodrama with looked after children and young people. *Dramatherapy*, 38: 2–3, 133–147.

Nairn, A and IPSOS MORI (2011) Child wellbeing in UK, Sweden and Spain: The role of inequality and materialism. Available via: https://www.unicef.org.uk/publications/ipsos-mori-child-well-being/.

Neil, E. (2019) Planning and Supporting Birth Family Contact when Children are Adopted from Care, Rudd Adoption Research Programme. Available at: www.umass.edu/ruddchair/sites/default/files/rudd.neil.pdf.

Newman, B. and Newman, P.R. (2018) *Development Through Life – A Psychosocial Approach*, (13th edn). London: Cengage Learning.

NHS (2019) Selective mutism. Available at: www.nhs.uk/conditions/selective-mutism/.

Noakes, A. (2019) Considering the risks to children of parental alcohol misuse. *Journal of Health Visiting*, 7:1. Published online: 22 January 2019, https://doi.org/10.12968/johv.2019.7.1.14.

O'Higgins, A., Ott, E.M. and Shea, M.W. (2018) What is the impact of placement type on educational and health outcomes of unaccompanied refugee minors? A systematic review of the evidence. *Clinical Child and Family Psychology Review*, 21, 354–361.

Panksepp, J. (2015) *The Neuroscience of our Emotional Lives*, paper given at the Conference at the Centre for Child Mental Health, London 26 April 2015.

Perry, B. and Szalavitz, M. (2008, reprinted 2017) *The Boy who was Raised as a Dog and Other Tales from a Child Psychiatrist's Notebook*. New York: Basic Books.

Bibliography

Peterson, A., Meehan, C., Ali, Z. and Durrant, I. (2017) What are the educational needs and experiences of asylum-seeking and refugee children, including those who are unaccompanied, with a particular focus on inclusion? A Literature Review. Canterbury Christchurch University. Available at: https://repository.canterbury.ac.uk/researcher/80x6z/mr-zulfi-ali.

Porges, S. and Daniel, S. (2017) Play and the dynamics of treating medical trauma: insights from Polyvagal Theory. In Daniel, S. and Trevarthen, C. (eds) *Rhythms of Relating in Children's Therapies*. London: Jessica Kingsley.

Raby, K.L. and Dozier, M. (2019) Attachment across the life span: Insights from adoptive families. *Current Opinion in Psychology*, 25, 81–85.

Robertson, E.K. and Gallant, J.E. (2019) Eye tracking reveals subtle spoken sentence comprehension problems in children with dyslexia, *Lingua*, 228. https://doi.org/10.1016/j.lingua.2019.06.009.

Sales, N.J. (2016) *American Girls: Social Media and the Secret Lives of Teenagers*. New York: Alfred J. Knopf.

Save the Children (2016) One girl under 15 married every seven seconds, 10 October 2016. Global. Available at: www.savethechildren.net/news/one-girl-under-15-married-every-seven-seconds.

Scolaro, E., Venkatraman, C-M, Khosla, R., Say, L. Temmerman, M., Blagojevic, A., Filion, B. and Svanemyr, J. (2016) *Child, Early and Forced Marriage Legislation in 37 Asia-Pacific Countries*. World Health Organisation and Inter-Parliamentary Union.

Sellers, R., Smith, A., Leve, L.D., Nixon, E., Cassell, J. and Harold, G. (2019) Using genetically informed research designs to better understand family processes and child development: Implications for adoption and foster care focused interventions. *Adoption and Fostering*, 43:3, 351–371.

Selwyn, J. (2019) Sibling relationships in adoptive families that disrupted or were in crisis. *Research on Social Work Practice*, 25:2, 165–175.

Sen, R. (2015) Not all that is solid melts into air? Care-experienced young people, friendship and relationships in the 'digital age'. *British Journal of Social Work*, 46:4, 1050–1075.

Shonkoff, J.P. and Levitt, P. (2010) Neuroscience and the future of early childhood policy: Moving from why to what and how. *Neuron*, 67:5, 689–691.

Simpson, J.E. (2013) Managing unregulated contact in the age of new technology: Possible solutions. *Journal of Adoption and Fostering*, 37:4, 380–388.

Simpson, J.E. (2016) A divergence of opinion: How those involved in children and family social work are responding to the challenges of the Internet and social media. *Child and Family Social Work*, 21:1, 94–102.

Sobel, D. (2017) Looked after children and attachment theory. *Headteacher Update*, 2017:2.

Stanley, N. (2011) *Children Experiencing Domestic Violence: A Research Review*. Totnes: Research in Practice.

Sunderland, M. (2015) *Conversations that Matter: Talking to Children and Teenagers in Ways that Help*. London: Worth Publishing.

Sutton-Smith, B. (1981) A History of Child's Play. Philadelphia: University of Pennsylvania Press.

Teicher, M.H., Samson, J.A., Anderson, C.M. and Ohashi, K. (2016) The effects of childhood maltreatment on brain structure, function and connectivity. *Nature Reviews Neuroscience*, 17, 652–666.

Twenge, J. (2017) *I Gen: Why Today's Super-Connected Kids Are Growing Up Less Rebellious*. New York: Atria (Simon & Schuster).

UNICEF (2018) Child marriage (updated April 2020). Available at: https://data.unicef.org/topic/child-protection/child-marriage/.

Van der Kolk, B.A. (2005) Developmental trauma disorder: Toward a rational diagnosis for children with complex trauma histories. *Psychiatric Annals*, 35:5, 401–408.

Van der Kolk, B.A. (2015) *The Body Keeps the Score: Mind, Brain and Body in the Transformation of Trauma*. London: Penguin.

Vidal, L. (2016) Developing innovative best practice solutions to address forced marriage in Australia. *Report to the Winston Churchill Memorial Trust of Australia, showcasing learning from Sri Lanka, UK, Denmark, US, Canada & Kenya*. Available at: www.researchgate.net/profile/Laura_Vidal17/publication/335014337.

Von Rege, I. and Campion, D. (2017) Female genital mutilation: Implications for clinical practice. *British Journal of Nursing*, 26:18, 22–27.

Warner, M. (2014) *Once Upon A Time…A Short History of Fairy Tale*. Oxford: Oxford University Press.

Waters L., Loton, D.J., Dawson, G., Jacques-Hamilton, R. and Zyphur, M.J. (2019) Observing changes over time in strengths based parenting and subjective wellbeing for Pre-teens and teens, Melbourne. *Developmental Psychology*. Available at: www.frontiersin.org/articles/10.3389/fpsyg.2019.02273/full.

West, G.L., Konishi, K., Diarra, M., Benardy-Chorney, J., Drisdelle, B.L., Dahmani, L., Sodums, D.J., Lepor, F., Jolicoeur, P. and Bohbot, V.D. (2017) Impact of video games on plasticity of the hippocampus. *Molecular Psychiatry*, 23, 1566–1574.

Willis, R., Dhakras, S. and Cortese, S. (2017) Attention deficit hyperactivity disorder in looked after children: A systematic review of the literature. *Current Developmental Disorders Reports*, 4, 78–84.

Winfield, C. (2019 2nd edn) *Gender Identity: The Ultimate Teen Guide*. London: Rowman and Littlefield.

Wing, L. (1996) *The Autistic Spectrum: A Guide for Parents and Professionals*. London: Constable.

Wood, J. (2020) Rethinking how we view gang members. An examination into affective, behavioural and mental health predictors for UK gang-involved youth. *Youth Justice online*, ISSN 1473–2254, University of Kent.

Woolgar, M. and Baldock, E. (2014) Attachment disorders versus more common problems in looked after and adopted children: Comparing community and expert assessments. *Child and Adolescent Mental Health*, 20:1, 34–40.

Zimbardo, P.G. and Coloumbe, N.D. (2012) *The Demise of Guys: Why Boys are Struggling and What we Can Do About It*. Amazon, Kindle edition.

Index

Index

Index